Robert Winslow Gardner

**Gardner's syrup of hydriodic acid**

therapeutical indications with clinical data

Robert Winslow Gardner

**Gardner's syrup of hydriodic acid**
*therapeutical indications with clinical data*

ISBN/EAN: 9783741190957

Manufactured in Europe, USA, Canada, Australia, Japa

Cover: Foto ©Lupo / pixelio.de

Manufactured and distributed by brebook publishing software
(www.brebook.com)

Robert Winslow Gardner

**Gardner's syrup of hydriodic acid**

# PREFACE.

For years letters have been constantly received from members of the medical profession representing that when Gardner's preparations are prescribed, others are substituted, from which failure results, causing great disappointment to the prescriber, and disaster to the patient.

Of late these complaints have increased to such an extent, coming as they do from all sections of the country, and the evil of substitution has now become so great that it cannot longer be borne.

The medical profession will give the writer credit for a strict regard to legitimacy during the twenty years and more that he has been engaged in preparing high-class pharmaceutical preparations for their use, confining his attention to those of which he has made an especial study. Every means at his command has been tried to prevent the abuse complained of. There is now absolutely no course left but the one decided upon, viz. :

Gardner's syrup of Hydriodic Acid will in the future be put up in 16 fl. oz., 8 fl. oz. and 4 fl. oz. bottles. Every cork will be covered by a strip label, bearing the manufacturer's signature in fac simile, and monogram seal (R. W. G.) in wax, uniting strip label to the bottle in such manner that it cannot be removed without destroying the integrity of the package.

Physicians desiring to prescribe Gardner's preparations can *rely upon having them dispensed,* if they will prescribe *original bottles* of a size to their requirements, and *specify Gardner's.*

It is sincerely hoped that by the adoption of these methods physicians will be enabled to procure these preparations when they so desire, be protected from substitution, and the vast mass of correspondence which has been heretofore required on this subject be no longer rendered necessary.

While Hydriodic Acid has long been known, it has not been possible to use it, as it could rarely be found in an undecomposed state until this syrup was made known. The text books have very little on the therapeutics of this remedy, except excerpts from literature written from professional experience in the use of Gardner's syrup. This pamphlet contains about all of this reproduced.

*All* papers published herein in their allusion to this remedy refer particularly to *Gardner's syrup* and *results obtained by it; not imitations of it.* The Clinical Index will afford opportunity for ready and quick reference by physicians to the various therapeutic applications of this remedy.

Probably no medicine in the whole *materia medica* has so wide a field of usefulness, or is administered in a greater number of diseases than that of iodine, and the voluminous reports of successful cases treated, which are embodied in this pamphlet, only emphasize this fact.

This is also confirmatory of the statement made in the editorial found elsewhere, that Gardner's syrup of Hydriodic Acid is not only the best form to administer iodine, when iodine is indicated, but is the best form by which it is *rapidly absorbed*—the thing most to be desired by the successful practitioner.

Among the many *new* applications, special attention is called to its great value in diseases of the genito-urinary system.

The very high standing of the professional men who have contributed papers upon this remedy, and the influential journals which have been the medium for such communications, should be noted.

During the extreme hot weather of summer syrup of Hydriodic Acid is occasionally decomposed.

This would not occur if it could be kept *cold* and corked. In such cases the manufacturer requests that the druggist *write*, informing him of the *exact amount*, and he will see that he *suffers no loss*.

Syrup of Hydriodic Acid is *good*, unless it has acquired an *orange* tint or darker. A light yellow is *not* a sign of decomposition.

Thankful for the appreciation with which my preparations have been received by the medical profession,

I am very truly yours,

R. W. GARDNER.

# SYRUP OF HYDRIODIC ACID.

## CLINICAL INDEX,

# LIST OF MEDICAL CONTRIBUTORS,

P. J. Bailey, M. D., Dawson, Ky.

C. E. Baum, M. D., Providence, R. I.

W. II. Bentley, M. D., LL. D., Cold Spring, Woodstock P. O., Ky.

Dr. Bauman, New Haven Hospital, New Haven, Conn.

W. R. D. Blackwood, M. D., Philadelphia, Pa.

W. D. Blatchely, M. D., Fort Scott, Kansas.

L. Bolton Bangs, M. D., New York City.

J. M. Blakesby, M. D., Germantown, Pa.

L. A. Briggs, M. D., Berlin Mills, N. H.

Leon De Bremon, M. D., The Late, Knight Leg. Honor, Mem. Ord. Imp., Ot. Medj., Mem. N. Y. County Med. Soc., Neurol Soc., Med. Legal Soc., late Clinical Assistant to Dr. Churchill.

E. S. Bunker, M., D., Late Prof. Obs. I. I. Col. Hosp., Brooklyn, N. Y.

F. A. Burrall, M. D., New York City.

John Cooper, M. D., Brooklyn, N. Y.

J. B. Carver, M. D., Fort Scott, Kansas.

James Craig, M. D., The Late, Jersey City, N. J.

J. K. Cantrell, M. D., Alton, Mo.

J. W. Daniel, M. D., The Late, Houston, Texas.

F. E. Daniel, M. D., Austin, Texas.

Walter M. Darnell, M. D., Belton, Texas.

C. L. Dodge, M. D., Kingston, N. Y.

D. C. DeWolfe, M. D., New York City.

F. F. Dickman, M. D., Fort Scott, Kansas.

A. U. Evarts, M. D., La Porte City, Iowa.

W. B. Fletcher, M. D., Indianapolis, Ind.

Henry M. Field, A. M., M. D., LL. D., Newtown, Mass., Lat. Prof. Ther. Dartmouth Med. Col.

F. R. Fraker, M. D., Marlboro, N. Y.

F. II. Garlock, M. D., Racine, Wis.

B. E. Gardner, M. D., Atlanta, Ill.

Malcom Graham, M. D., Jonesville, Mich.

Allen McLane Hamilton, M. D., N. Y. City, Prof. Dis. Mind and Nerve System, N. Y. Polyclinic.

Stinson Harrison, M. D., Washington, D. C.

James Lewis Howe, M. D., Louisville, Ky., Dean Hos. Col. Med. and Sur.

C. F. Huddleston, M. D., Troy, N. Y.

William F. Hutchinson, M. D., The Late, Providence, R. I.

E. P. Hurd, M. D., Newburyport, Mass.

William Judkins, M. D., Cincinnati, Ohio, Late Prof. Phys., etc., Col. Med. and Surg.
J. M. Keller, M. D., Hot Springs, Ark.
Ferdinand King, M. D., New York City.
F. John Kaufman, M. D., Syracuse, N. Y.
Charles H. Knight, M. D., New York City.
Charles Lengel, M. D., Kansas City, Mo.
J. II. Lennon, M. D., Little Rock, Ark.
Louis Lewis, M. D., F. R. C. S., Philadelphia, Pa.
S. T. Lowrie, M. D., Lore City, Ohio.
I. N. Love, M. D., St. Louis, Mo., Prof. Dis. Child., Clinical Med. and Hygiene
    Marion Sims Col. Med.
Thomas H. Manley, M. D., New York City.  Phys. to Harlem Hosp. Surg. Clinic.
S. C. Martin, M. D., St. Louis, Mo., Prof. Derm. and Hygiene, Barnes Med. Col.
Charles K. Mills, M. D., Philadelphia, Pa., Prof. Mental Dis. and Med. Juris. Univ.
    Penn., Neurologist to Philadelphia Hosp.
L. S. Nicholson, M. D., Washington, D. C.
J. P. Oliver, M. D., Boston, Mass.
Joseph M. Patton, M. D., Chicago, Ill., Prof. Intern. Med. Chicago Polyclinic.
Louis G. Pedigo, M. D., Crockett Springs, Va.
W. T. Peyton, M. D., Louisville, Ky.
William Porter, A. M., M. D., St. Louis, Mo., Phys. to Prot. Hosp., St. Luke's and
    City Hospitals.
A. Rose, M. D., Lebanon, Ky.
John V. Shoemaker, A. M., M. D., Philadelphia, Pa., Prof. Skin and Ven. Dis., Med.
    Chir. Hosp., Phys. to Phil. Hosp. for Dis. Skin, &c.
Logan Stanley, M. D., Fincastle, Ind.
C. C. Stephenson, M. D., Little Rock, Ark.
Q. C. Smith, M. D., Austin, Texas.
A. Springer, M. D., Lewiston, Me.
II. F. Stowell, M. D., Rochester, N. Y.
Richard II. Taylor, M. D., Hot Springs, Ark.
James J. Terhune, M. D., Brooklyn, N. Y.
W. S. Todd, M. D., The Late, Ridgefield, Conn.
L. A. Turnbull, M. D., St. Louis, Mo., Visiting Phy. to Fem. Hosp., St. Louis, Mo.
W. J. Weischelbaum, M. D., Savannah, Ga.
Conrad Wienges, M. D., Jersey City, N. J.
W. C. Wile, A. M., M. D., LL. D., Danbury, Conn.
James A. Williams, M. D., New York City.
John W. Williamson, M. D., Boydton, Va.
J. C. Willson, M. D., Morley, N. Y.     ·
J. T. Wrightson, M. D., Newark, N. J.
W. Gill Wylie, M. D., New York City.
T. J. Yount, M. D., Lafayette, Ind.
I. Burney Yeo, M. D., F. R. C. P., London, England.   Prof. Clin. Therap., King's
    Col. Hosp. and Auth. "Man. Med. Treat. or Clin. Therap."

WORLD'S COLUMBIAN EXPOSITION,

Chicago, 1893.

———

# GARDNER'S

# SYRUP OF HYDRIODIC ACID

Received Medal and Diploma

## OF THE FIRST CLASS.

# ONLY AWARD

Granted Syrup of Hydriodic Acid Over all
Competitors to

## R. W. GARDNER, of NEW YORK.

## Administration of Iodine.

# GARDNER'S

## Syrup of Hydriodic Acid.

Iodide of Hydrogen.                                      Non-Irritant Iodine.

Syrup of Hydriodic Acid, as prepared by R. W. Gardner, is a clear, white or very slightly yellowish-tinted syrup, of a pleasant sub-acid taste, reminding one of lemon syrup. It contains 6.66 grains of iodine in each fluid ounce, or 6.712-1000 grains gaseous Hydrogen Iodide (HI,). *Hydrogen Iodide consists of 99.22-100 parts of Iodine, and 78-100 of one part Hydrogen.*

Iodine, probably the best alterative of the *materia medica*, strange to say has been heretofore administered in its least available forms, namely, in those chemical combinations in which the iodine retains its irritant and caustic character.

The most frequently employed form is that of iodide of potassium, a combination of two irritant substances, iodine and potassium.

The irritant action of iodine is not at all modified by its combination with potassium, but on the contrary is rendered more so, by the added acridity of the base.

Lugol's solution contains free iodine; iodide of iron contains iodine in an irritant condition, but this is not usually noted, because of the infinitesimal proportion contained in the dose, hence iodide of iron is a better means of administering iron than iodine. Iodide of sodium is only less of an evil than iodide of potassium, as both elements retain their caustic properties. Causticity and irritation are not the only objections to iodides of potassium and sodium; these bases combine with and neutralize the hydrochloric acid of the gastric juice, which being necessary to digestion, this process is interrupted, and the appetite fails, producing depression and loss of nutrition, in addition to the constitutional difficulty for which the iodine is pre-scribed. The longer iodide of potassium is continued, the worse these effects become, until in many cases, the remedy must be discontinued to allow the patient to recover from the condition caused by the remedy.

The advantages of Hydriodic Acid (iodide of hydrogen,) as a means of administering iodine, need merely to be stated to be enthusiastically endorsed.

Natural secretions are aqueous; water consists of hydrogen and oxygen; hydrogen is therefore a natural element and component of the liquids of the body, the solvent of substances absorbed and elim-inated. Hydrogen is therefore a natural base and superior to all others for combination with substances designed for assimilation.

Iodide of Hydrogen (Hydriodic Acid,) is non-irritant, has an acid re-action and consequently does not interfere with digestion, is more active than iodide of potassium, is as palatable as lemon syrup, may be given freely to delicate women and young children, and may be continuously used, without intermission, (except in cases where iodism occurs,) until the full effects of the iodine are produced, and the morbid state corrected. It produces no depression, indiges-tion, nor irritation. It is indicated whenever iodine is required for internal use.

Hydriodic Acid possesses all the antiseptic properties of iodine, all its alterative action. Its use as an internal antiseptic is one of its most remarkable applications. Being absorbed so promptly that it is detected in the urine in ten minutes after administration upon an empty stomach, having in this short time passed through the circula-tion, it will at once be seen that as an internal antiseptic it must be invaluable. No other form of iodine is so freely tolerated, hence the antiseptic action of iodine as an internal remedy, has not been here-tofore available. All diseases of an infectious character, and all septicæmic conditions, cannot fail of improvement under this remedy. Being non-irritant, and tolerated to the point of saturation of the system, it promises to become the ideal internal antiseptic that the profession has been so long searching for.

In forming an estimate of the therapeutic value of Hydriodic Acid, it should be borne in mind that it differs materially from iodide of potassium in its chemical composition; inferences from the observed effects of the potassium salt, its relative strength in iodine, and even its therapeutic action, must, consequently, be modified by a consideration of the difference in chemical composition, and hence, in therapeutic action.

The therapeutics of Hydriodic Acid were practically unknown until 1878, (excepting Dr. Wylie's experience,) as no *permanent* form of it was available. Clinical experience since then, has demonstrated that it is much more effective than potassium iodide, more easily and pleasantly absorbed, and is capable of producing results, and being used in cases, impossible with iodide of potassium.

The observed effects of its administration in syphilis, for instance, when if the potassium salt is used, it is usually considered necessary to administer it in large quantities to obtain the desired results, seems to point to a great difference in activity between the two forms of iodine, in favor of Hydriodic Acid.

Hence, hasty conclusions, drawn from experience with iodide of potassium, and calculating the relative therapeutic value of Hydriodic Acid from the comparative iodine strength of the two compounds, will, undoubtedly, be found erroneous.

Hydriodic Acid is a distinct remedy by itself, and should not be handicapped by the observed effects of another form of iodine, different in composition and action.

Small doses, in syphilis, according to the experience of many physicians, produce such desirable results, that it is reasonable to conclude, that Hydriodic Acid, because of its different chemical form, its greater activity, and more assimilative character, is much more efficient, and may be capable of producing, in small doses, and with no disturbance to the system, all the results which have heretofore required heroic doses of potassium iodide, with the inevitable production of the unpleasant symptoms usual in such cases.

Dr. W. Gill Wylie, the eminent specialist of New York City, first suggested to the writer the great desirability of having a permanent form of Hydriodic Acid, that could be relied upon by physicians. The doctor himself, and his father, also a practicing physician of Chester, S. C., had previously used an extemporaneously prepared form of the remedy with advantage.

Acting upon the suggestion of Dr. Wylie, after much experiment, the present Gardner's syrup of Hydriodic Acid, was perfected and put on the market, and the result of its use by him appeared in a paper by Dr. W. Gill Wylie, April, 1879. (Page 29.)

It has been demonstrated beyond peradventure to the minds of some of our ablest practitioners, that Gardner's syrup of Hydriodic Acid is the ideal antiseptic of the *genito-urinary tract*. This statement can be easily verified by you, by testing it in the very next case of pyelitis or chronic cystitis among 'the many that constantly besiege you for relief. There are probably few sufferers who pass such wretched lives as those who are continuously tormented with vesical irritation, and any remedy that will afford relief and permanently benefit the condition, will be hailed as a boon by physicians and patients alike.

Prof. J. H. Lenon, M. D., Little Rock, Ark., January, 1894, mentions three cases of enlarged prostate gland, treated with syrup of Hydriodic Acid, with satisfactory results.

A case of enlarged prostate gland, in an old gentleman over eighty years of age, has been reported by Dr. John W. Williamson, of Boydton, Va., January, 1894. He writes: "When the syrup was. first given, about two months ago, the patient was compelled to void his urine every two or three hours, and then with difficulty. He could not retain it without suffering much pain about the neck of the bladder and prostate. Now he voids not oftener than every six to eight hours, and could retain it longer, if prudent to do so, without pain. The stream is more normal, and there is much less. difficulty in micturition. The absence of pain on retention indicates less irritability, and the stream shows less enlargement or hypertrophy of the gland. There was thought to be a complication of slight subacute cystitis."

In commenting on the effects of this remedy, Dr. Williamson continues: "It must be a most valuable reconstructive and alterative tonic for the nervous system, and therefore has much influence on the various secretions and organic functions. It keeps the bowels perfectly regular and normal in action, improves appetite and digestion, and, indeed, general improvement of the whole system."

**Uric Acid Diathesis.**—Dr. Ferdinand King, of New York city, reports a case of uric acid diathesis, (stone) entirely cured by Gardner's syrup of Hydriodic Acid.

On the seventh of December, 1893, Dr. King writes as follows: "I prescribed your syrup of Hydriodic Acid in a case of chronic nephritis five days ago, and the patient reported to-day. 'All symptoms have disappeared.' This convinces me that it is the remedy, par excellence, for diseases of the kidneys caused by excess of uric acid. I want the profession to know what syrup of Hydriodic Acid will do in kidney troubles. A trial in these cases will convince the most skeptical."

Dr. W. C. Wile, Danbury, Conn., calls attention to the value of syrup of Hydriodic Acid in the kidney pain which accompanies pyelitis and renal colic. This pain will be recognized as being more or less severe, quite constant, aggravating and sleep-destroying, particularly after active exertion. It was prescribed for the doctor, by L. Bolton Bangs, M. D., the eminent authority on genito-urinary diseases, of New York. Dr. Wile's paper will be found on page 73.

**Pyelitis and Cystitis.**—In *Pyelitis and Cystitis* this remedy has evidently a grand future before it. A case reported by Dr. W. B. Fletcher, of Indianapolis, Ind., is truly remarkable, resulting in a perfect cure of both conditions.

The case was one of ten years' standing. Dr. Fletcher's paper will be found on page 70. (See also case of chronic cystitis treated by Dr. J. M. Blakesby, Germantown, Ky., page 66.)

**Cataract.**—An elderly lady had been operated upon for cataract. Both eyes affected, but one, only, operated upon; the sight was still quite obscure. She had at this time an attack of chronic bronchitis, to which she was subject, for which she was advised to take Gardner's syrup of Hydriodic Acid. Shortly after commencing its use she was surprised to find that her eyesight was rapidly improving; this improvement continued and remained permanent. The oculist had arranged for a second operation, (needling,) but found her condition such that it was unnecessary. Doubtless the operation, in this case, had much to do with the improvement, but the fact that a sudden change for the better occurred upon the use of the Hydriodic Acid syrup, and that a subsequent operation became unnecessary is strong proof of its utility in causing absorption of the cataract.

The other case was that of an old gentleman, who had made an engagement with his oculist for an operation for cataract, and for whom his regular physician had prescribed Gardner's syrup of Hydriodic Acid for other troubles; he, also, was much surprised to observe a marked improvement in his sight; this, in his case, could not be attributed to any other cause than the syrup, as he had not taken any other medicine, and the oculist had not yet treated him. The operation had been postponed.

Later reports from this case are to the effect that the cataract has not progressed, that the operation has not yet been found necessary, though the sight is not restored. Still there has been improvement. The case being far advanced and the patient about eighty years of age, at the time the treatment was commenced, and the fact that some improvement has been observed, instead of progress in the cataract is favorable to the action of the remedy.

It would naturally be inferred from the history of that case that the cataract would be completely dissolved if treated in the incipient stage. Thus it will be noted, it makes an advance in the therapeutics of this intractable malady. In confirmation, Dr. D. C. DeWolfe, one of the visiting surgeons of the Manhattan Eye and Ear Hospital, New York city, reports two cases of traumatic cataract, with most marked improvement when under the influence of the syrup of Hydriodic Acid.

While the final result in these two cases has not yet fully developed, the influence of this remedy has shown such marked progress that it naturally leads to the conclusion that it is an advance on former methods. The doctor promises to report these cases in extenso, as soon as the permanent results are obtained.

Hydriodic Acid being a powerful antiseptic and resolvent, is a special stimulant to the activity of the secretory system of glands.

It favors rapid elimination of debris. The uric acid diathesis is an essentially septic condition, not only in the kidneys and appendages, but throughout the entire organism.

An efficient internal antiseptic which will act without producing irritant or toxic effects has long been desired.

Iodine stands at the head of alteratives, and as a result of the persistent administration of this remedy you get tissue metamorphosis or change, combined with its antiseptic action, upon an organ like the uterus, which is composed almost entirely of elastic muscular tissue, permeated in every direction by a vast net work of blood vessels. It also produces in this organ the same as it does in the kidney, a soothing effect upon the nerves supplying it, through some process which as yet is not capable of explanation. While theoretically it is impossible for the physician to explain the physiological action of many of the most important remedies which he uses in his daily practice, abundant clinical experience, as in this case, goes to prove beyond question its value. You have here either an active or passive congestive condition, according to whether the inflammation is acute, sub-acute, or chronic. The capillaries are more or less gorged with blood. It is a well-known clinical fact that the dilatation of the capillaries produces the pain that accompanies, in a greater or less degree, every form of inflammation. It is also a well-known fact that iodine under these conditions produces a contraction of the capillaries, lessening the tension and reducing pain.

While we do not present this as a positive explanation, still it is very reasonable to suppose that this is its action. Dr. A. Rose, Lebanon, Ky., says: "There is a wide field of usefulness for this preparation that so far has been little dreamed of," referring to his gynæcological experience in the treatment of tubal disease of the ovary, leucorrhœa and dysmenorrhœa. (Page 55.)

**Chronic Bronchitis.**—Every physician practicing north of Mason and Dixon's line, and many south of it, will acknowledge that the most harassing feature in chronic bronchitis is the pronounced, prolonged and frequent cough, due to the effort of the patient to expel the tough, thick, tenacious, stringy mucus ever present in this disease.

The result of these continued efforts is far out of proportion to the substance raised.

Its clinging character, close to the bronchial walls, while causing constant irritation and desire to cough, forces the patient to great expulsory effort. This almost continuous and violent exercise sooner or later exhausts the patient to such a degree that the general tone is impaired and the healthy standard reduced. It is in reducing this cough and rendering expectoration easy that we find one of the most valuable and pronounced results from the administration of syrup of Hydriodic Acid. It takes but a little while after the commencement of the treatment for the patient to discover, with a sense of relief and satisfaction, that a slighter effort is required to bring up a much larger quantity of mucus. This is due, first, to the direct therapeutic action of the syrup on the mucous membrane of the bronchi, in an increase of the secretion; second, on account of the alterative and antiseptic action of the syrup, fully explained elsewhere, this secretion is much thinner and of a much less viscid character, and underlying the old, tenacious mucous which is ever present, clogging every tube, renders expectoration easier, with less effort—a thorough cleaning out of the tubes is the result—and an increased air space rendered available for the better and more rapid oxygenation of the blood.

As a result of this treatment, then, we get easier expectoration, less sustained muscular effort at expulsion, general improvement of the health, and, finally, the ultimate cure of the disease which so stubbornly resists the best applied therapeutics. This effect, relieving the congestion of the mucous membrane, is well illustrated in the treatment of croup. Paper by Dr. Stinson Harrison, Washington, D. C., page 52. Also in general catarrhal affections, when the secretion is offensive, they become innocuous, "acting as a disinfectant as much as many of the remedies which have been placed on the market for that purpose." (Dr. Garlock's paper, page 53.)

In chronic bronchitis, the experience of the following physicians will be of interest:

John V. Shoemaker, A. M., M. D., Philadelphia, Pa., page 30; W. C. Wile, A. M., M. D., LL. D., Danbury, Conn., page 32; F. H. Garlock, M. D., Racine, Wis., page 53; Franklin Jno. Kaufman, M. D., Syracuse, N. Y., page 65; T. J. Yount, M. D., Lafayette, Ind., page 39; James A. Williams, M. D., New York City, page 61; Chas. Lengel, M. D., Kansas City, Mo., page 63; J. Stinson Harrison, M. D., Washington, D.C., page 52; Henry M. Field, A. M., M. D., Newtown, Mass., page 44; and numerous others whose writings can be found in the Clinical Index, page 6.

**Poisoning by Lead, Mercury and Arsenic.**—Hydriodic Acid affords the best means of treating poisoning by lead, mercury and arsenic, as the iodine converts the metal into the iodide, a soluble form, in which it is taken up by the secretions and eliminated from the system. It is better than potassium iodide for this purpose, as it can be continued until the desired result is obtained without causing depression, or interfering with digestion. (Paper by W. C. Wile, Danbury, Conn., page 32.)

**Bronchial Asthma.**—Dr. W. Gill Wylie, of New York, and Dr. J. P. Oliver, of Boston, were the first to call attention to the efficacy of this remedy in these affections. It is now considered by those who have used it, as affording more speedy, thorough, and complete relief in these cases than any other remedy.

If specimens of some of the letters which have found their way to the writer, from laymen suffering with asthma, who, snatched from the horrors of suffocation by the use of this syrup, prescribed by the attending physician, could be seen, it would do more to convince the profession than any remarks of mine.

Of course letters from laymen are not available. They have reached me through the physician telling his patient what he has prescribed, and in the gratitude of their hearts they have expressed their feelings in personal letters. While the best proof of its usefulness is a personal test, I would refer the reader to papers by Dr. W. Gill Wylie, New York, page 29, Dr. Oliver, Boston, Mass., page 34, Henry M. Field M. D., Newtown, Mass., page 44, J. W. Daniel, M. D., Houston, Texas, page 64, James A. Williams, M. D., New York City, page 61, Louis Lewis, M. D., F. R. C. S., Phila., Pa., page 58.

**Hay Fever.**—This troublesome affection, is so wide-spread, and distressing to the patient, so obstinate to treatment, requiring the sufferer to actually flee from his home, and spend long seasons in localities free from its baneful influence, will, in most cases, yield to treatment by syrup of Hydriodic Acid. In this disease, as in grippe, the cause is doubtless a germ, which becoming located in the nasal passages and trachea, produces the constant irritation characteristic of the disease. Acting as a germicide upon the microbe, the cause is eliminated, while by stimulating the entire mucous surfaces to increased secretion, the congestion and inflammation are relieved.

The evidence is very strong, as given by prominent practitioners. The reader is referred to an article by William Judkins, M. D., late professor of physiology, etc., Cincinnati College of Med. and Surgery,, page 39, and John V. Shoemaker, A. M., M. D., Phila., Pa., page 30, and S. C. Martin, M. D., St. Louis, Mo., page 71.

**La Grippe and Sequelæ.**—The antiseptic properties of syrup of Hydriodic Acid, are especially useful in this disease, doubtless acting as a germicide upon the spirillæ in the organism, reducing temperature, and preventing, if used in time, the obstinate bronchial cough which accompanies the disease. (Paper by Dr. C. L. Dodge, Kingston, N. Y., page 58.) In the sequelæ from grippe, certain nervous disorders are sure to follow.

Dr. L. A. Bridges, Berlin Mills, N. H., reports his experience in these cases, where everything else failed, complete relief followed the use of this syrup. (Page 53.)

**Pulmonary Catarrh, Chronic Accumulations of Serous Fluid.**—Dr. Henry M. Field, late professor of therapeutics in Dartmouth Medical College, has written an exhaustive paper upon syrup of Hydriodic Acid. He divides his subject, treating first of its chemical characteristics; second, of dispensing, care and preservation, ingestion, &c.; third, the physiology of its action; and fourth, of its therapeutics, in which he gives high praise to its action in the above complaints. (Page 44.)

**Goitre, Exophthalmic.**—Syrup of Hydriodic Acid stands at the head of remedies for this affection, and cases are constantly reported of cures of the worst cases.

In the *Reference Hand-Book of the Medical Sciences*, page 765, Allen McLane Hamilton, M. D., Professor of Diseases of the Mind and Nervous System, N. Y. Polyclinic, in an article on goitre, says: "I have used galvanism with good effects, but rely almost entirely upon a little known remedy, Hydriodic Acid, with which I have cured three cases of advanced and serious goitre. This is given in aqueous solution (Gardner) in increasing doses."

Dr. W. C. Wile, of Danbury, Conn., reports a severe case cured by it. (Page 33.)

Dr. J. B. Carver, Fort Scott, Kansas, reports (page 51) two cases, one of which was desperate, the heart's action being so tumultuous that the entire body vibrated, and she could not stand still.

Dr. W. B. Fletcher, Indianapolis, Ind., reports a very severe case. "Eye-lids could not be closed completely. Pulse, 130 to 140. Breathing difficult." (Page 56.)

Dr. W. Gill Wylie, New York, strongly recommends it in goitre, and chronic malarial poisoning. (Page 29.)

**Acute Inflammatory Rheumatism.**—This is one of the most important applications of this remedy.

The late Dr. Jas. Craig, of Jersey City first called the attention of the medical profession to its value in this disease, pointing out that under this treatment the heart is free from complications, the remedy preventing the exudation and organization of plastic material.

Under the syrup of Hydriodic Acid the duration of the disease is shortened, relieving pain and reducing temperature in a much shorter time than by other measures. It should be given at once, without regard to the fever, and pushed, that the alterative action be obtained in the least possible time. (Papers by Jas. Craig, M. D., Jersey City, N. J., page 35 to 38.)

W. J. Weischelbaum, M. D., Savannah, Ga., page 66; Lewis G. Pedigo, M. D., Crockett Springs Sanatarium, Va., page 49; W. C. Wile, A. M., M. D., LL. D., Danbury, Conn., page 32; J. W. Daniel, M. D., Houston, Texas, page 64; J. H. Garlock, M. D., Racine, Wis., page 53 and 54, and others. (Clinical Index.)

**Chronic Rheumatism.**—In the chronic form of the disease the relief will be just as sure, though from the nature of the case, much more time will be required for the remedy to eliminate the waste products which have become permanently located in the organism in an insoluble state, and which are the cause of the condition. It will frequently be found that the resolution of these substances, uric acid and other products of destructive metabolism, which are ever present in this disease, will be accompanied by an exacerbation of pain for a short period, followed by corresponding relief. The fixation of joints and contraction of muscles, will slowly but surely yield to the treatment. The fact that the Hydriodic Acid acts as a diuretic, as well as an alterative gives it a peculiar advantage in this condition. T. J. Yount, M. D., Lafayette, Ind., page 65; Chas. Lengel, M. D., Kansas City, page 63; Lewis G. Pedigo, M. D., Crockett Springs.

:Sanatarium, Va., page 49; W. T. Peyton, M. D., Louisville, Ky., page 67; J. W. Daniel, M. D., Houston, Texas, page 64.

**Scrofulous Diathesis.**—In this connection it is unnecessary to say more than refer to the well known value of iodine as an alterative. As to the practical evidence of the power of this syrup in these cases, the instances are so numerous and results so satisfactory, that I merely refer to papers by J. W. Daniel, M. D., Houston, Texas, page 64; John V. Shoemaker, M. D., Philadelphia, Pa., page 30; Dr. Nicholson, Washington, D. C., page 65; W. C. Wile, A. M., M. D., LL. D., Danbury, Conn., page 32, etc. (Clinical Index.)

**Suppurative and Subsequent Stages of Small-Pox.**—A convincing proof of the internal antiseptic value of Hydriodic Acid is given in the paper of Dr. W. H. Bentley, Woodstock, Ky., (page 43.) The Doctor used it in the suppurative and subsequent stages up to complete desquamation, in an epidemic, treating thirty-one cases—all made complete and rapid recoveries.

**Acute Pneumonia.**—Dr. Bentely also reports twenty-three cases of acute pneumonia treated with syrup of Hydriodic Acid "always with good results" (page 41.) See also paper by, J. Stinson Harrison, M. D., Washington, D. C., page 52.

**Chronic Pleurisy and Sequelæ of Acute Pleurisy.**—Dr. Lewis G. Pedigo, Crockett Springs, Va., gives a history of his own case; he was under treatment by eminent authorities in New York, and was told he would be compelled to winter in the south and leave his practice. But under the action of this syrup, he not only continued his practice, but to the surprise of his physicians and himself, it was found that he had so far recovered, that the advice was reconsidered and he was allowed to stay.

Later, being examined by a careful physician for life insurance, to whom he gave a history of his case, and mapped out the location of the old trouble, he was told after thorough physical examination, that no local evidence of adhesion or other morbid condition could be discovered. (Page 49.)

**Specific and Non-Specific Urethritis.**—If syrup Hydriodic Acid posseses the antiseptic properties which seem to be demonstrated by the authorities quoted, it would appear to be adapted to the treatment of such infectious and inflammatory conditions as the above.

Clinical experience shows that iodide of potassium in this class of cases has a powerful influence, especially in those of a specific or scrofulous diathesis. This being true, it follows as a matter of course that iodine is the curative agent and the syrup of Hydriodic Acid being the best form of administration, must prove of value to the practitioner who meets with this class of intractable cases. It is suggested that in patients in whom there is a suspicion of either of these taints, that this remedy be given a faithful test.

**Strumous, Syphilitic, and Tuberculous Diathesis.**—Dr. Thos. H. Manley, New York, at his surgical clinic, Harlem Hospital, says, that syrup of Hydriodic Acid is the ideal way of exhibiting iodine. He always uses it in preference to any other remedy, to tone up the system in persons of strumous, syphilitic or tubercular tendencies, before operations. "Indeed, in most cases, its timely and appropriate employment would obviate the necessity of any sort of surgical interference."

**Definite Iodine Strength.**—In a preparation of this character, relied upon for important therapeutic effects, it is of the first importance that it shall be uniform in composition, as otherwise invaluable time is lost in the treatment, during which the disease may progress with serious results to the patient. It is also necessary that the remedy shall produce its results with the least disturbance to the system.

The late Dr. William F. Hutchinson, the eminent specialist in nervous diseases, speaking of syrup of Hydriodic Acid, says: "When medicine must be continued indefinitely, as in some cases of sclerosis or neuritis, in small, unvarying quantities it must be in such form as will not disturb digestive organs or become physically disagreeable." After alluding to the unpleasant effects of potassium iodide, in producing violent coryza, hoarseness, sore throat, etc., he says: "Gardner's syrup has changed all that. It is agreeable to the eyes, taste and stomach, non-irritant to mucous membranes." "I find that this preparation is by far the best form of iodine for rapid dosing, as it is pleasant to taste and rarely, if ever, produces coryza."

Dr. F. F. Dickman, Fort Scott, says: "Too much credit cannot be given Mr. Gardner in keeping this preparation up to a standard

of excellence and purity found in none of the numerous imitations
that are found in the shops. In fact, we have found that almost
invariably, when failure of beneficial results are reported, that some
other manufacturer's product has been dispensed. It is unfair to
blame the drug or decry it as worthless, unless a good article has been
used. We know Gardner's syrup to be an excellent remedy, and
when recommending the preparation we mean the original Gardner's
syrup, and not an imitation." (Page 67.)

Not to mention too many of such statements here, the reader is
referred to expressions by numerous other physicians, whose opin-
ions on this point are emphatic, and will be found throughout the
clinical literature published herewith.

**Fibroma.**—Dr. H. F. Stowell, Rochester, N. Y., reports: "A
case of fibroid tumor in the region of the parotid gland of twenty
years' duration.

A perceptible shrinkage occurred during the first two months of
treatment by syrup Hydriodic Acid, after which it remained
stationary. There was, however, total relief of various unpleasant
sensations in the growth, which sometimes amounted to pain. An
inveterate *eczema* (life long) entirely disappeared. (Page 58.)

Dr. James A. Williams, New York, reports a fibroid tumor of
the breast, size of an orange, in. a lady aged 40 years. After three
months' treatment with syrup Hydriodic Acid, she had gained 25
pounds in weight and scarcely a trace of the tumor remained.

Another case reported by the same physician, two tumors (variety
not stated), one on the neck and one on the side; the one on the
neck is all absorbed, the one on the side three-fourths gone; is feeling and looking finely and has gained 15 pounds in weight. (Page 61.)

Dr. James J. Terhune, Brooklyn, N. Y., reports seven cases of
uterine fibroids cured by syrup of Hydriodic Acid. (Page 72.)

The late W. S. Todd, M. D., Ridgefield, Conn., reports a case
of uterine fibroid treated with complete recovery.

Dr. Weischelbaum, Savannah, Ga., reports a case of fibroid
tumor treated with syrup of Hydriodic Acid with good results.
(Page 66.)

Dr. W. Gill Wylie, New York, reports a case of adipose tumor,
relieving the pain and reducing the weight of the body. (Page 29.)

**Typhoid Fever.**—Dr. B. E. Gardner, Atlanta, Ill., (page 66) writes: "Whenever I get a dry, red tongue, or in typhoid fever, I use it, and always get good results."

**Eczema.**—Dr. F. E. Daniel, Austin, Texas, says: "Gardner's syrup of Hydriodic Acid, has a wide therapeutic range, but its most brilliant powers are brought out in eczema, that protean disease, which so baffles the doctor, and in scrofula." (Page 67.)

Dr. John V. Shoemaker, Philadelphia, Pa., the celebrated authority and author of a text-book on skin diseases, recommends it in eczema, particularly in children. (Page 30.)

Dr. F. R. Garlock, Racine, Wis., strongly recommends it in chronic eczema, not of specific nature; in cases complicated with syphilitic taint, it is all that could be desired, if used simultaneously with usual mercurials. (Page 53.)

Dr. W. C. Wile, A. M., M. D., Danbury, Conn., also recommends it in infantile eczema. (Page 32.)

**Lupus.**—Dr. W. H. Bentley, Cold Spring, Woodstock, Ky., reports a case of two years' standing, and two inches in diameter, situated on the left leg of a woman, thirty-two years old. At the expiration of seven weeks it was reduced to the size of a twenty-five cent piece. Later she reported herself entirely well. (Page 40.)

**Spinal Disease.—Obscure.**—The importance of remedies which change the condition of the blood, in chronic diseases, brought on by a depraved or impoverished state of this "living tissue," is frequently overlooked in an attempt to relieve prominent local symptoms by stimulants and tonics, which are not useful as blood makers, or depuratives.

The late eminent specialist, Wm. F. Hutchinson, M. D., of Providence, R. I., relates the history of a case of obscure spinal disease, which will illustrate the remarks made above. (Page 57.)

**Syphilis.**—"Probably the greatest value to the practitioner of syrup of Hydriodic Acid, will come from its employment in syphilis, particularly in the latter stages. The stomach is often rebellious at this time, for it has most likely been surfeited with mercury. Many cases drag along under iodine, because not enough of it can be borne, and mercurials are frequently, not only useless, but at times injurious. Instances such as those related bear admirably, large doses of syrup of Hydriodic Acid. Some cases have come under my observation in which the patients were at a stand still, who at once brightened up and rapidly improved under the use of the syrup of Hydriodic Acid. If thought desirable, the biniodide of mercury, (the red salt) can be combined with the syrup." John V. Shoemaker, A. M., M. D., Phila., Pa. (Page 30.)

This view of the efficacy of Hydriodic Acid in syphilis, is only what would naturally be expected from this admirable form of iodine, as its great assimilability, non-irritant character, and *direct* and *prompt* action as an alterative in other conditions has been proven.

Dr. A. Rose, Lebanon, Ky., says: "I have tested it in all forms of syphilis—primary, secondary, and tertiary. In the latter there are but few manifestations of the disease after having used the remedy. The secondary symptoms are held in abeyance, until it is convenient to administer a few steam and mercury vapor baths; when the further use of the mercurial plaster, and a continued use of Gardner's syrup of Hydriodic Acid, every physician may hopefully and confidently expect the happiest results to follow at once. I have used it in syphilis, when anæmia was marked, when potassium iodide, iodide of iron or mercury in any form could not be tolerated one moment; anæmia disappeared, the continuous headache instantly ceased, sore throat got well at once, all glanular swellings disappeared. The gummata everywhere vanished into thin air, and the irruption was held in statu quo, until I could give a few calomel vapor baths." (Page 55.)

Richard H. Taylor, M. D., Hot Springs, Ark., relates a case where iodide of potassium could not be borne. Cured with not only success, but in a remarkably *short* time. (Page 52.)

In phthisis with syphilitic complications, the paper by Dr. William Porter, of St. Louis, Mo., will be interesting and instructive. (Page 59.)

As an evidence of the wide spread reputation, which syrup of Hydriodic Acid has attained in the medical world, I. Burney Yeo, M. D., F. R. C. P., London, Professor clinical therapeutics, Kings College Hospital, in his "Manual of Medical Treatment or Clinical Therapeutics," vol 1, page 534, says: "The syrup of Hydriodic Acid, made by Gardner, of New York, is largely used in America, as a substitute for potassium iodide in the treatment of asthma, chronic bronchitis, and other diseases in which the use of iodine is indicated."

**Myelitis.**—Charles K. Mills, M. D., Professer of mental diseases and Medical Jurisprudence, University of Pennsylvania, Neurologist to Philadelphia Hospital, in the "International Clinics," fourth series, page 100-101, says: "One of the best combinations of drugs in the early stages is probably that of the iodides" and further on in the latter stages.

"Now use tonics, as strychnine, and every thing to improve the nutrition of the patient; and alteratives such as syrup of Hydriodic Acid may prove useful."

**Purpura, Sclerosis of Liver.**—Two cases reported by Dr. J. K. Cantrell, Alton, Mo. "Child two and one-half years old, most successfully treated of any case attended during a twenty years' practice. The case of sclerosis of liver rapidly improving. Had hæmoptysis until almost dead. No hemorrhage since taking the remedy." (Page 69.)

**Obesity—Fatty Degeneration of the Heart.—Amyloid Liver.**—Dr. F. A. Burrell, New York, mentions a case of enlarged liver, supposed to be amyloid, in which the gland diminished as shown by measurement under this syrup. He considers it a valuable remedy in glandular enlargements, obesity and fatty degeneration of the heart. (Page 61.)

**Dosage.**—This remedy should usually be given half hour before meals.

No absolute rule can be laid down for dosage, as this must be regulated according to the conditions.

As a general guide it may be said that doses will vary from one-half teaspoonful to one teaspoonful, always diluted with two table-spoonfuls of water.

In hay fever, asthma, chronic bronchitis, catarrhal affections, and where the object is to relieve local inflammatory conditions, it is better to begin with small doses, say half a teaspoonful in water, and gradually increase until the alterative action upon the mucous surfaces has given the desired relief. If iodism is produced, reduce, intermit, or suspend the remedy, and resume its use when the symptoms have subsided.

In acute rheumatism, the remedy may be given without regard to the fever, at intervals of two to four hours, in doses varying from a teaspoonful to a tablespoonful, until pain is relieved, which is usually in from twenty-four to forty-eight hours, and then gradually discontinued.

In this acute inflammatory disease it is desirable to obtain its full physiological action in the shortest time; it should, therefore, in these cases, be given in doses as large as can be borne, and thus secure by its rapid assimilation the greatest benefit as soon as possible.

In syphilis, the remedy is to be pushed according to the symptoms and toleration of the patient, until the condition is controlled.

As has been said elsewhere the effect of Hydriodic Acid is more prompt and active than that of iodide of potassium and, probably, much smaller relative doses will be found effective, than usually employed when iodide of potassium is used in this disease.

# CLINICAL EXPERIENCES WITH SYRUP OF HYDRIODIC ACID.

## A SUBSTITUTE FOR IODIDE OF POTASSIUM.

### BY W. GILL WYLIE, M. D., NEW YORK CITY.

(Reprinted from the *N. Y. Medical Record*, May 10, 1879.)

Seven years ago, while with my father, at that time practicing in Chester, S. C., I found that he was using Hydriodic Acid in place of iodide of potassium. The case that suggested its use was one of asthma; for many years the patient had suffered from this troublesome affection. Whenever she contracted an ordinary cold, it would extend to the chest and cause at once persistent asthma, which, if left to itself, would last for weeks. A full dose of morphia would relieve the spasmodic and labored respiration, and large doses of iodide of potassium would remove the bronchitis in a short time. Often the iodide would irritate the stomach and seriously interfere with digestion. To get the best effects it was necessary to give from fifteen to twenty-five grains of the iodide, three times a day, Hydriodic Acid was prepared by mixing one drachm of iodide of potassium with ninety grains of tartaric acid, and dissolving in four ounces of water. On trial, it was found that one teaspoonful of this mixture had as much influence on the bronchial surfaces as twenty grains of iodide of potassium, and produced no bad effect whatever on the stomach. The only difficulty was, that the simple solution soon decomposed and set free the iodine; to obviate this it was mixed with a very heavy syrup, and when properly prepared it made a clear solution which could be kept several days without showing much sign of decomposition.

Gaseous Hydriodic Acid (HI) is rapidly and perfectly absorbed by water, but being held by a feeble chemical affinity, the hydrogen soon becomes disengaged, and sets free a corresponding amount of iodine, which, being soluble in Hydriodic Acid, passes into solution, colors it red, and renders it too irritating for internal use.

As 100 parts of Hydriodic Acid consist of 99.22-100 parts of iodine and 78-100 of a part of hydrogen, it will be seen that it is nearly all iodine, and when not decomposed it is entirely non-irritant and pleasantly acid to the taste. To make the syrup it requires care, and most drug shops will get up sufficient decomposition in the mixing to render the solution useless.

Several months ago, I sent for R. W. Gardrer, of New York, whose syrups of the Hypophosphites I had used with much satisfaction, and suggested that he would try and prepare a syrup of Hydriodic Acid. He succeded in making a syrup containing forty minims of the dilute acid to the ounce representing 6.66-100 grains of iodine, which corresponds to 8.69-100 grains of potassium iodide, which keeps perfectly. Two teaspoonfuls of syrup is an average dose.

I have had some patients that could not take even very small doses of iodide of potassium, or iodine in any form, without producing severe iodism. Some of these cases gave distinct accounts of active poisoning, others seem to have the idiosyncrasy show itself with the first dose of iodine. Other patients easily bear twenty-five grains potasssium iodide, three times a day, for weeks at a time. In the use of Hydriodic Acid I have seldom found it necessary to increase the usual dose to get the desired effect. It would seem that iodide of potassium becomes active by being coverted into Hydriodic Acid.

For the past six years, I have had uniformly good results in the use of Hydriodic Acid in bronchitis, and in chronic and sub-acute catarrhal diseases. I have found that it acts as an irritant, and does more harm than good during acute febrile stages. I have also used it in chronic malarial poisoning, and in Graves' disease, and would recommend its use in the place of iodine in goitre and adipose tumors. In a case of the latter, it relieved the dull pain about the tumor and reduced the weight of the body slightly (the patient being very fleshy.)

I have not used Hydriodic Acid in syphilis long enough to give an opinion as to its value in this disease.

The text-books on therapeutics do not even mention Hydriodic Acid, and the *National Dispensatory*, edited by Alfred Stillé, M. D., and John M. Maisch, Ph. D., says: "Pharmaceutically, Hydriodic Acid is a very unsatisfactory preparation." "It possesses no medicinal value."

---

## HYDRIODIC ACID.

### By JOHN V. SHOEMAKER, A. M., M. D., PHILADELPHIA, PA.

(Reprinted from the *Medical Bulletin*, August, 1889.)

If any alterative is more in demand than the iodides, it would puzzle therapeutists to agree upon its name. Many obscure deviations from health exist, amounting not only to pronounced disease, which will not give way to simple tonics or to depurants of the purgative order. These maladies are the bane and torment of a busy doctor, and many times he gets them out of his list by the use of iodides. Then again, when well-defined cases of scrofula and syphilis are under our care, the value of a good alterative is pre-eminently a question of moment. Unfortunately, the iodides in large or long-continued doses have a tendency in many instances to inaugurate stomach disorders, and yet the absolute need of the remedy is apparent. What then shall we do? We can have recourse to Hydriodic Acid. For years this agent was officinal in the dispensatory, but it was dropped because of its unstable character, which made it not only unpleasant, but unsafe to administer. For almost ten years the acid was not obtainable, until in 1878, when Mr. R. W. Gardner, of New York, introduced the agent in the form of a syrup, which the best tests have shown to be unalterable by any ordinary exposure in the sick room, unless in hot weather, when, of course, it should be excluded from either extreme light or heat. Sufficient time has now elapsed to demonstrate that the claims made for the syrup are well founded, and that it replaces the salts of soda and potassa in an entirely satisfactory manner. An important addition in the form of the syrup of Hydriodic Acid has therefore been made to current therapeutics. By the use of this syrup we obtain, in a palatable form, iodine in its most effective state. Mr. Gardner has shown that:

\* \* \* \* \* \* \* \* \*

Its effect upon mucous surfaces is more marked than with other forms of iodine, while it is effective in smaller relative proportions, and when required, it is so free from irritant action that it may be given to the youngest infant. \* \* \*

The syrup of Hydriodic Acid is especially serviceable in asthma, hay fever, acute and chronic rheumatism, chronic bronchitis and in many chronic congestions of the mucous tract. Probably the greatest value to the practitioner of syrup of Hydriodic Acid will come from its employment in syphilis, particularly in the latter stages. The stomach is often rebellious at this time, for it has most likely been surfeited with mercury. Many cases drag along under iodine because not enough of it can be borne, and mercurials frequently are not only useless, but at times injurious. Instances such as those related bear admirably large doses of syrup of Hydriodic Acid. Some cases have come under my observation in which the patients were at a standstill, who at once brightened up and rapidly improved under the use of the syrup of Hydriodic Acid. If thought desirable, the biniodide of mercury (the red salt) can be combined with the syrup, but the protiodide cannot be used at the same time, because it (the green salt) would be converted into the former salt, and unless care was taken the unexpected activity of the syrup thus prepared would exceed the prescriber's expectations, and possibly injure the patient. In syphilis the syrup can be pushed, if needed, until the characteristic saturation is evident, or when the metallic taste becomes pronounced, and we know that iodism is near at hand. It is advisable, however, not to carry the administration so far.

In rheumatism the syrup may substitute the alkalies and may cut acute attacks short sooner than the ordinary drugs that are usually prescribed. It is certainly a useful article in chronic muscular rheumatism. It has done good service in my hands in sciatica. It may be administered during acute rheumatic attacks without reference to the fever, and in moderate doses, say a teaspoonful or two every two hours. Of course, it will not act promptly and effectually in all cases, for rheumatism is notoriously fickle as related to curative agents. In bronchial disorders small and frequently repeated doses are better than large ones. It may be administered in this latter affection in from twenty to thirty drops every two hours. The syrup has been recommended in chronic arsenical poisoning, several cures being noted. In lead poisoning it has also been serviceable. In obesity the steady administration of the syrup of Hydriodic Acid with suitable regimen has a very happy effect. We are not too well supplied with agents of repute in this disagreeable complaint. Hence a note on this point in reference to its use in this respect is of utility.

Many skin diseases are benefited by the syrup of Hydriodic Acid. In connection with cod liver oil it is valuable in some varieties of eczema, particularly in children. It is especially efficacious in the form known as scald head, which is often so obstinate and unyielding to many remedies. Scrofulous persons (those predisposed to glandular troubles) receive decided benefit from its use. The red-eyed children, those having recurrent granular lids, with repeated attacks of mild conjunctivitis, derive great relief from syrup of Hydriodic Acid. A case of amyloid liver with fatty heart, in the practice of Dr. F. A. Burrall, of New York, was notably aided by the syrup of Hydriodic Acid, and he endorses it in glandular troubles generally. Dr. Blackwood, of Philadelphia, has employed it largely in his practice, and reports cases of exophthalmic goitre, lumbago and uterine catarrhs which were cured by the syrup. It is desirable that Hydriodic Acid should be given by itself, inasmuch as it is very susceptible to chemical action, combinations with other remedies might act injuriously upon it. Metals and alkalies are incompatibles, so also are oxidizing agents, as for instance, acids, permanganate and chlorate of potassium. These would form iodic acid, which would be highly injurious to the patient. If intolerance becomes apparent, as occurs with all really active medicines after a more or less extended use, the syrup should be dropped for a week or ten days, when most likely the stomach will have recovered its tone and it may again be administered. Unlike many remedies which, when once objected to in this way, are never likely to be good again, the syrup is just as palatable and equally efficient when taken up after a vacation (so to speak) as when first given, which is an important characteristic of this remedy. Although syrup of Hydriodic Acid is used by many practitioners, we call attention to it, believing that a wider knowledge of it is desirable and feeling certain that a careful trial by physicians at large will add to their armamentarium an important remedial agent, as they will learn to appreciate its value as we have, by its employment in a wide circle of disease for many years.

# HYDRIODIC ACID—ITS USES IN GENERAL PRACTICE.

## By WM. C. WILE, A. M., M. D., LL. D., DANBURY, CONN.

Ex-Vice-President of the American Medical Association, Member of the British Medical Association, Editor of the *New England Medical Monthly*, etc., etc.

Read before the American Medical Association, Cincinnati, 1888.

The difficulties which were in the way of the use of Hydriodic Acid because of its rapid decomposition were considered so insurmountable that it was not until the year 1880, when an unalterable syrup was presented to the profession, that it came into use. Soon after this, in 1880, my attention was attracted to an article by Dr. J. B. Oliver, of Boston, which was published in the *Boston Medical and Surgical Journal* of the issue of March 4th of that year.

Dr. Oliver, in his paper, alluded to the use of syrup of Hydriodic Acid in the treatment of asthma, and, in conclusion, says that Dr. Knight "had surprisingly satisfactory results" from the same remedy. Having under observation at this time a severe case of chronic asthma, complicated with chronic bronchitis, on which I had tried iodide of potassium, which was intolerable to the stomach, I at once put the lady, a woman of forty-nine years, upon the syrup of Hydriodic Acid. The effect was all that could be desired. There was an almost immediate relief from the asthmatic conditions, rapid amelioration of the cough, decreased expectoration, which was very profuse before the exhibition of the remedy. The sputa, which was thick and viscid, became thinner in character, and my patient's general health commenced to improve, and after three months of the use of the syrup of Hydriodic Acid, in increasing doses, till two teaspoonfuls were taken, three times a day, complete recovery took place, and from that time till her death of pneumonia, two years later, had no relapse. The results in this case were *so* satisfactory that ever since it has been my favorite remedy in *all* asthmatic troubles, and though every case has not yielded so promptly and effectually as this one, still I have never administered it in this class of diseases without unmistakable evidences of relief and comfort. In chronic bronchitis of long standing in my hands it has produced most excellent results, and can be given when the iodide of potassium cannot for a moment be tolerated. The cases which seem to derive the most benefit from this remedy belong to that class of long standing bronchitis, when the lung seems about to take on a deeper seated and less tractable form of disease. My attention has been frequently called, in the treatment of chronic bronchitis with Hydriodic Acid, to the fact that small doses, frequently repeated, are of signal service, when larger doses do not seem to accomplish the same results. In fact, from long experience, I would suggest the constant use of the syrup in small doses, fifteen drops, gradually increased a drop a dose, until the point of toleration is reached, in order to get the most satisfactory and lasting results. While practicing at Sandy Hook, Conn., I had the opportunity of observing its action in lead poisoning in a great many cases, lead entering largely into the compound which is mixed with the crude rubber during the process of manufacture. I depended almost entirely on the syrup of Hydriodic Acid for all forms of chronic lead poisoning. In lead paralysis this remedy, combined with keeping the bowels quite free, and the application of the faradic current, were the only means employed, and always with satisfactory and oftentimes surprising results.

Wrist-drop and chronic abdominal pains would yield to the remedy, combined with saline cathartics. In scrofulous diseases, of children especially, does the Hydriodic acid seem to produce most marvelous results. In infantile eczema, enlarged glands, cold abscesses, indolent sores, treated with small doses, gradually increased until it is all that can be borne, will prove a source of great gratification to the patient and gratitude toward the doctor.

At the suggestion of my friend, Dr. F. A. Burrall, of New York, I am using it in a case of obesity, with the result of steady diminution of the amount of fat, without a single disagreeable symptom, or interference with the general health, or the actions of any of the functions of the body. In hay fever it has been used by other observers with good results, but my own experience with its use in this disease has been *nil*.

It is hardly necessary for me to more than say that in all the latest stages and manifestations of syphilis it has yielded its most magnificent results. Pleasant to take rapidly pushed to large doses, I have found the most pronounced and favorable effects. Patients take it readily, and the improvement is so rapid and immediate that they need no urging to continue its use for as long a time as the doctor deems desirable.

My paper has now reached the limits which I prescribed for it, but I cannot resist the temptation of recording briefly three of the most unique cases of my experience with this drug. The one was a man, forty-two years of age, who was a paper box manufacturer, suffering from arsenical poisoning from the inhalation of arsenical dust arising from the glazed paper which he handled and cut. After repeated trials of other remedies, the syrup of Hydriodic Acid made a complete cure inside of a month.

In Danbury, the city in which I now reside, they make large quantities of hats; in fact, it is said that at least one-half of the hats made in the United States are made in that place. To preserve the fur, carrot is used, which is composed largely of mercury; consequently, many of the hatters working in the plank shop suffer from mercurial poisoning, and many from mercurial tremor and paralysis. No remedy has proved of so much value to me as the Hydriodic Acid, always prompt in its effect and reliable in its results. The last case was one of chronic rheumatism in a man thirty-seven years old. He was almost a complete cripple in his hands and feet and had not done a stroke of work in two years. I had exhibited every remedy known to me, including electricity, massage, Turkish baths, colchicum, etc., etc., etc., but until I commenced the use of the Hydriodic Acid no permanent improvement was made. After continuing its use for four months the patient seemed, and was to all appearances entirely well. For fear of relapse, he continued taking it for two months more, in order, as he explained it, "to make assurance doubly sure." I do not believe that this remedy is enough understood for the advantages it possesses over all other forms of iodine nor as thoroughly appreciated as it should be, but of this I am assured, that it will be tolerated by the stomach many times when no other preparation of its class can be retained, and do work that none other will. It is scarcely necessary for me to state that I have never used any other preparation than that of the originator of the syrup, Mr. R. W. Gardner, of New York.

---

# A CASE OF GOITRE CURED BY GALVANISM AND SYRUP OF HYDRIODIC ACID.

By WILLIAM C. WILE, A. M., M. D., LL. D., DANBURY, CONN.

(Reprinted from the *New England Medical Monthly*, November, 1892.)

Cases of exophthalmic goitre; while not very common, are not infrequently met with by the general practitioner. I do not remember of seeing over eight or nine in a large practice of twenty-three years. A large proportion of the cases, usually met with and usually treated as laid down in the text books, rarely fully recover. So when one meets with a case which has entirely recovered by a course of treatment, it is his duty to make it known to his brother practitioners.

The case which I shall now narrate, is only a prototype of many such cases, and the interest is not in the novelty of the treatment [for it is an old one] but from the fact that it got well inside of eight months, and by simple measures.

Mrs. B., thirty-seven years old; American. Mother of four children; resident of

Brooklyn, N. Y., consulted me January 17, 1892, for what she believed to be heart disease. She had always been perfectly well up to three months previous, then she had a very severe attack of "La Grippe." Pneumonia arose as a complication and she came near losing her life. Her convalescence was long and tedious, and as soon as she commenced to move around, she noticed a good deal of palpitation of the heart. Food did not digest well, and when she did eat, the irregular action of the heart was increased, till oftentimes she would be compelled to lie down, which seemed to relieve her. Any unusual exertion, sudden shock, or excitement would produce violent and rapid pulsations. Slept badly; and was so nervous, that, as she expressed it, "she felt like flying out of her skin."

She thought that she had organic disease of the heart. A physician had told her so, and she thought she was liable to die at any time. She was emaciated, and in a miserable condition, generally, unhappy herself, and making every one else unhappy about her.

A careful examination revealed the fact that there was no organic disease of the heart; that the nervousness, and the palpitation were due to a commencing Graves' disease. She had the enlargement of the thyroid gland, exophthalmia, notably of the left eye, and all of the nervous phenomena of commencing exophthalmic goitre.

I regulated the bowels, put her on a plain nourishing diet, gave her sulfonal gr. xxx at bedtime every night and then every other night for a while, to make her sleep.

Administered from eight to ten cells of the galvanic current, placing the positive pole inside the left ear, and the negative over the seventh cervical vertebra, applying the current for twenty minutes daily.

Internally, syrup of Hydriodic Acid [Gardner's] was given, commencing with teaspoonful doses three times a day, gradually increasing the dose till two tablespoonfuls was at one time taken, t. i. d.; then was again reduced to a teaspoonful, when it was stopped at the end of seven months.

The improvement was immediate and rapid. The galvanism was stopped at the end of a month, and for six months she continued to use the syrup of Hydriodic Acid till the 23d of September when I discharged her, perfectly cured.

## THE TREATMENT OF ASTHMA.

### By J. P. OLIVER, M. D., Boston, Mass.

(Reprinted from *Boston Medical and Surgical Journal*, March 4, 1880.)

In Dr. F. I. Knight's review of Berkart on asthma, he incidentally alludes to the results of my treatment of asthma with large doses of iodide of potassium. In connection with the above, I desire to state that the drug, in doses of five or ten grains, seldom gave relief; but large doses, continued for a long period, gave entire relief in the majority of cases. Some patients however, were unable to take the iodide of potassium even in small doses; in such cases, I used, as a substitute, Hydriodic Acid, and, as Dr. Knight says, 'with surprisingly satisfactory results.' The form I have oftenest used is the syrup of Hydriodic Acid, and that prepared by Robert W. Gardner, of New York, I consider the best; it is agreeable to the taste, and not very likely to be affected by exposure to light and air. It should be given as follows: Begin with small doses, twenty or thirty drops well diluted with water, and taken about half an hour to an hour before meals; if taken after meals, it may disturb the stomach, set up fermentation, and cause colic. acid stomach, and pain in the head; increase the dose gradually, and a tablespoonful dose should not be exceeded. In cases of chronic bronchial catarrh, and in fact in all cases where iodine is indicated, I have found the syrup of Hydriodic Acid of great value.

Later in the season, I propose to send to the *Journal* a report of a large number of cases of asthma treated on the above plan, and with very gratifying results.

## ACUTE INFLAMMATORY RHEUMATISM.

BY THE LATE JAMES CRAIG, M. D., JERSEY CITY, N. J.

(Reprinted from *New York Medical Record*, April 21, 1883, page 448.)

Before using the remedy shortly to be spoken of, I was in the habit of prescribing bicarbonate of potassa, which, as a rule, gave relief as soon as the urine was rendered alkaline, which required about a week or ten days, and during that time opiates had to be given to relieve pain and produce sleep. I have also prescribed salicylic acid, but cannot say that I have seen any decided benefit from its use.

Syrup of Hydriodic Acid, prepared by Robert W. Gardner, of New York, is the remedy *par excellence* for this painful and troublesome affection.

I have used it for the past two and a half years in bronchitis and scrofula, but its effects have been most prompt in acute inflammatory rheumatism, relieving pain in from twelve to forty-eight hours.

I have been called to see patients suffering from this affection, and found them with high fever, joints swollen, and suffering terribly, and on the following day have been agreeably surprised at their rapid improvement, finding them in a great measure free from pain and fever reduced. Some other cases take a longer time, but I have yet to find one that was not in comfortable condition within forty-eight hours.

The dose I prescribe for *adults* is from two to three teaspoonfuls, every two or three hours, in a wineglass of water, until relieved; afterward I reduce the dose to one teaspoonful, which may be continued for five or six days, at longer intervals.

I was first led to the use of this remedy in prescribing for a patient suffering from bronchitis complicated with rheumatism, its effects being most salutary in the relief of both diseases.

I should state that under this mode of treatment, the heart has been free from complications; the remedy preventing exudation and organization of plastic material. I more frequently use it now in rheumatism than in bronchitis; in fact, I use it in all cases of acute rheumatism, and must say have always been pleased with its results. I have also prescribed it in chronic rheumatism, but with less effect. I hope that other physicians will give it a fair trial, and find it as useful in their hands as it has been in mine.

---

## NOTES OF SIXTEEN CASES OF ACUTE RHEUMATISM.

BY JAMES CRAIG, JERSEY CITY, N. J.

(Reprinted from the *New York Medical Journal*, August 8, 1882.)

In an article appearing in the New York *Medical Record*, April 21, 1883, I speak of the manner in which I was led to the use of this syrup in cases of acute inflammatory rheumatism. The object of the present article is not merely to reiterate what is said in that publication, but to emphasize my entire faith in the efficacy of this treatment by the citation of cases of cure, and the statement that I have yet to find a case in which, the syrup being properly used, it has failed to meet my expectations.

Since the publication of my first article this method of treatment has been employed by a number of physicians with success, shortening the duration of the disease, relieving pain, reducing temperature, and in all cases leaving the patient without heart complications, the remedy preventing exudation and organization of plastic material. I order the syrup in from two to three teaspoonful doses, in a wineglass of water, every two hours, lessening the dose as improvement takes place, and continuing the syrup for about a week or ten days after the symptoms have disappeared, to insure recovery and prevent relapse.

· The old method of treatment by the use of bicarbonate of potassium is slow, and its continued use brings about a depraved condition of the system by reducing the amount of fibrin in the blood and destroying the red corpuscles. It also acts as a irritant to the stomach, injuring the mucous membrane and causing loss of appetite. The depraved condition of the blood can be seen in the pale face, pallor of the lips, and enfeebled action of the heart, requiring weeks for the patient to recover from the disease and its treatment. Salicylic acid has had its day and has been found wanting, being replaced by some with oil of gaultheria—salicylic acid in another form.

This acid, from its difficult solubility, allows its chrystals to irritate the throat and stomach, and in some occasions so much vomiting as to render its continued use impossible.

Syrup of Hydriodic Acid is a good remedy in subacute rheumatism also, but is not so prompt in its action as in cases of the acute form.

I have tried it in chronic rheumatism, but cannot say that I have observed any good results. In some cases I use a lotion as follows:

R    Liq. plumbi subacetatis, 3 ij.
     Tincturæ arnicæ, ℥ ij.
     Aquæ, ℥ vj.

M. Sig. Add one part of the solution to three parts of hot water, and apply saturated flannels to the inflamed joints. It usually gives immediate relief. This solution is of a beautiful yellow color when properly prepared.

The following are a few of the numerous cases of successful treatment of inflammatory rheumatism by the use of the syrup of Hydriodic Acid:

CASE I. On December 16, 1880, I was called to see Mary S., aged eight years, who was suffering from a very severe attack of rheumatism. The knees and ankles were very much swollen, and the pain was so excruciating that she could not bear the weight of a sheet to touch her legs. Protected them with a barrel hoop cut in two and crossed. Prescribed syrup of Hydriodic Acid, in teaspoonful doses, every two hours. The pain was subdued within fifteen hours. Continued treatment for about a week. No relapse.

CASE II. Mrs. E. P. R., aged thirty-five years, was seized with a chill on January 9, 1883. Began the use of syrup of Hydriodic Acid on the 10th, and continued the treatment, in three teaspoonful doses, diluted with water, until the 16th, when the patient was dismissed cured.

CASE III. Mrs. C. F. C., aged thirty-nine. I was sent for on March 21, 1883, and found her suffering from acute rheumatism; prescribed the syrup in two teaspoonful doses; continued treatment to the 29th, when I made my last visit, and found my patient dressed, sitting up, and free from pain.

CASE IV. B. E., aged fifty-five, a merchant, has had rheumatism for many years. I attended him with a sub-acute attack on the 13th of January, 1884; left him on the 18th, free of pain. The medicine was given in tablespoonful doses, every two hours, up to this time, when he was ordered to continue its use in smaller doses and at longer intervals for another week. On the 4th of April, 1885, I was called to attend him with a similar attack. Used the syrup. The pain was still severe on the 5th, so I used the lotion to his hand and knee, which gave immediate relief. The last visit was made on the 8th, at which time he was entirely free of pain and swelling.

CASE V. Mrs. L. A., aged twenty-seven, was taken with a chill, followed with high fever, on the 21st of January, 1885. I was called on the 22nd, and found her suffering with an attack of acute rheumatism, affecting both upper and lower extremities. As usual in such cases, prescribed the syrup in three teaspoonful doses, every two hours, using the lotion as well. She was relieved in thirty-six hours, and was about the house in one week. Ten days after I made my last visit, her husband told me that she had had a relapse from imprudently sitting by an open window. Medicine was repeated, and in four or five days she was again free from pain.

CASE VI. W. C., aged twelve years, of stout build, was seized with rheumatism in knee, ankle and hand. Saw him for the first visit on February 20, 1885. I prescribed the syrup in two teaspoonful doses, diluted in water (which should always be done); the lotion was also used in this case. My last visit was made on the 28th, when I left him walking about the house.

CASE VII. S. G. S., aged thirty-eight, clerk, was seized on the morning of the 15th of March, 1885. Commenced the use of the syrup on the evening of the same day; he was free of pain and swelling on the 16th and went to his business on the 17th. He has had no return.

CASE VIII. J. C., aged fifty-one, has had chronic rheumatism for more than twenty years. About the beginning of March, 1885, he was seized with a violent pain in right knee, while walking, followed, after a few days, with heat and swelling. The affected knee was two inches larger in circumference than the other; the trouble was looked upon as a sprain for about three weeks, when rheumatism was suspected. Began the use of the syrup in tablespoonful doses in a gill of water; he felt relief after the second dose; treatment was continued every two or three hours until eight ounces of the syrup were taken; which removed all further trouble. No relapse.

CASE IX. John L., aged forty, coachman, was taken down on May 4, 1885; his knees were very much swollen and very painful. He was given the syrup in tablespoonful doses every two hours, and was able to be around the house in four days and a half. He had a relapse on the 24th of the same month, caused by exposure, and was seized with a chill, and again used the syrup and lotion. Advised the syrup to be continued in decreasing doses and at longer intervals for a week or ten days.

CASE. X. J. II., aged forty, conductor. I was sent for on May 29, 1885, and found his right knee and left ankle swollen and very painful. He also complained of pains in his fingers and toes. The syrup was given, in tablespoonful doses, every two hours; the lotion was also used. He was free from pain within forty-eight hours. Dismissed him on the 3d of June without pain or ache.

The following cases were kindly furnished me by my friend, Dr. Conrad Wienges, of this city.

CASE I. August 28, 1883. P. M., engineer, aged forty-nine; sub-acute rheumatism in both knees and ankles. Gave him two teaspoonfuls of syrup of Hydriodic Acid every three hours. Dismissed him September 3d, free from pain or ache. This patient had several attacks previous to this one, but was always confined to the house from four to six weeks.

CASE II. June 16, 1884. Mrs. L., aged thirty-five; sub-acute rheumatism in the chest and right shoulder. Two teaspoonfuls of syrup of Hydriodic Acid every four hours. It relieved the pain entirely in twenty-four hours.

CASE III. March 30, 1883. F. McC., nineteen years old; worker in tobacco factory; acute rheumatism in both knees and ankles. He was ordered two teaspoonfuls of syrup of Hydriodic Acid, every two hours, in wineglass of water. At my next visit, on the 31st, he could flex his knees and move his foot with comparative ease. April 1st, the swelling had vanished, and the patient was sitting up when I called. He was dismissed on the 3d, cured, and resumed his occupation on the 3d of April.

CASE IV. May 7, 1885. G. E. P., thirty years old; deck hand; acute rheumatism affecting the right shoulder and elbow. The pain was excruciating—so much so that one-fourth of a grain of morphia was given to produce temporary relief. He took two teaspoonful doses of Hydriodic Acid every two hours. At my next visit, sixteen hours later, the pain had almost disappeared, and he could move the arm with ease in any direction. On the 9th, he was entirely free from pain, and was dismissed cured on the 11th.

The following cases were kindly furnished me by Dr. Bauman, House Physician at the New Haven Hospital, New Haven, Conn.

CASE I. M. F. M., Irish, aged twenty-five; single; painter. Was attacked April 24, 1885, with acute rheumatism in the ankles and knees, and on the 25th it extended to his shoulders, elbows and wrists. Entered hospital this day; temperature 103° F. The pain was so severe that the slightest movement caused great distress. No cardiac lesions. Ordered syrup of Hydriodic Acid, one teaspoonful every two hours.

**38**

**28th.** Patient has improved greatly. Temperature 100°; joints not so painful.
**29th.** Improvement continues. Patient got up to-day.
**May 4th.** He is up and around the wards, and has no pain in his joints. Treatment continued.
**5th.** Discharged cured.
**CASE II.** P. M., aged twenty-two years. Has been under treatment in the surgical ward since April 28th, for gluteal abscess. Has had an attack of rheumatism in both wrists and hands, and pain in the chest and back. The pain and swelling was so severe that he could not bear to be touched. Temperature 100°. Ordered salicin, 20 grains, every three hours, and sodii bicarb., one-half drachm, every three hours.
**May 30th.** No marked improvement, and was transferred to medical wards. Salicin was stopped, and he was given syrup of Hydriodic Acid, two teaspoonfuls every two hours. Temperature 101.6°. Morphine, hypodermically, had to be administered during the night on account of severe pain.
**31st.** Pain diminished; morphine not required. Temperature 101.2°.
**June 1st.** Patient slept well without the use of anodynes. Fingers could be moved without pain, but chest was still painful.
**2d.** Patient comfortable; all pain and inflammation have disappeared. He fed himself for the first time to-day. Temperature 100°.
**5th.** He was transferred to the surgical ward, and syrup stopped.
**8th.** Temperature rose to 100.3°, and another attack threatened. He was given the syrup in the same doses. Next day temperature fell to normal. The syrup was continued a week and then gradually diminished and stopped.
**Remarks.**—The patient had previously had several attacks of rheumatism, each lasting from two to four weeks. He had a mitral regurgitant murmur on admission.

The syrup was tried in a number of sub-acute cases with good results, but was unsuccessful in chronic cases.

I hope that I have thus been able to impress upon the minds of my readers the fact that, by the use of the syrup of Hydriodic Acid in cases of acute inflammatory rheumatism, our results will be far more satisfactory, and our cases less tedious and uncertain.

---

## ASTHMA AND CHRONIC BRONCHITIS.

### By PROF. GERMAIN SEE,

In the translation of a lecture delivered in the "Hospital la Charite," Paris, on "Respiratory Medicaments," under the subject Iodine, occurs the following foot-note by the translator, E. P. Hurd, M. D., Newburyport, Mass.

(Reprinted from the *New York Medical Record*, Jan. 20, 1893, page 58.)

"A very good preparation containing iodine, much employed in this country, and especially commended for its palatableness, is the syrup of Hydriodic Acid. * * * It is sold through all the United States, and is in much repute as a remedy for asthma and for chronic bronchitis. The preparation which is most frequently prescribed in this region, is Gardner's syrup, which is certainly an elegant preparation, and has been given both in spasmodic and bronchial asthma, with very satisfactory results. Two teaspoonfuls is an average dose. Children take this syrup readily. It never irritates the stomach."

**Asthma.**—John Cooper, M. D., Brooklyn, N. Y., Nov. 14, 1893, writes: "It may be satisfactory for you to know that in the treatment of asthma, (free from heart lesion and purely depending upon spasmodic action of the fibres of the bronchi), much beyond my expectation, a curative effect has resulted from the use of your syrup of

Hydriodic Acid, and cannot but think that its use, if more generally known by the profession, would be found to accomplish that which other remedies only tend to palliate."
**Chronic Bronchitis.**—T. J. Yount, M. D., Lafayette, Ind., in the *New York Medical Record*, Aug. 4, 1893, page 121, writes: "Gardner's syrup of Hydriodic Acid, a non-irritant preparation, has a decided curative effect on this disease. I have used it on myself and many patients, and have experienced almost immediate benefit by the arrest of the profuse secretions and cough. The only objection to it is the strong and pronounced metallic taste which invariably follows its prolonged administration, causing loss of appetite and consequent debility. It should be given in teaspoonful doses three times a day at the commencement. and gradually increased to two or three teaspoonfuls three times a day, well diluted in Burgundy wine or water." * * * *

---

## HAY ASTHMA.

### BY WILLIAM JUDKINS, M. D.,

Late professor Physiology, etc., Cincinnati College Medicine and Surgery, Cincinnati, O.

(Reprinted from the *New York Medical Record*, Sept. 6, 1884.)

"**Hay Asthma—Can it be relieved?**"—I feel that I should be sadly derelict of duty did I not give to the profession, and through them to the laity, my successful treatment of this obstinate and distressing complaint. Though only the record of one case, the result is so gratifying to the patient, her family, and myself, that I feel justified in sending these few lines regarding it, in hope of benefiting others. Mrs. ——, aged twenty-eight, married, mother of two children, the youngest four and a half months old, has been subject to annual attack of hay fever for fourteen years, and frequently with complications of a severe character. Last year she suffered an attack of bronchitis, during the latter part of the asthmatic stage, that came near proving fatal. Convalescence slow. The case first came under my charge in 1880. The attack that year was aggravated in a measure by pregnancy. The only thing at that time that gave any relief was "'milk punch," in the proportion of whiskey 2 oz.; milk 8 oz. The relief obtained from this was only temporary, when more would be administered; but at no time was intoxication produced, though the remedy was given for several days in succession. In 1881, a reputed "hay fever resort," (Oakland Md.) was tried for a part of the season, but no benefit was derived, the attack being fully as severe as at any previous time. 1882 and 1883 were equally bad, the complication of bronchitis spoken of coming on last year, which almost caused death. This year phophylactic treatment was commenced, some two weeks before her expected attack, of valerianate of zinc, 1 gr., and pill asafœtida co., 2 gr., combined in capsules, one morning and afternoon, as recommended by Dr. Morrell Mackenzie, of London. It disagreed with her stomach, and was discontinued for three days, and then again taken with no bad effect. For five days after her usual time for the appearance of the dreaded affection all was serene.

The night of the 20th inst., difficulty of breathing to a limited extent set in. My attention had been called to a case of bronchial asthma which obtained relief from the use of Hydriodic Acid, and I immediately ordered my patient to commence its use early on the morning of the next day, the 21st. The effect, in conjunction with counter-irritation in the shape of Riggollot's mustard leaves at the wrist-joints, *was simply magical;* breathing became more and more easy as she continued the remedies. A thunder storm came up that night, twelve hours after commencing the medicine, and for half an hour she was somewhat "stuffed up," as she expressed it, but had a good night's rest. Ever since then she has been easy—now a week—but is exercising all precautionary measures against taking cold, for fear of relapse.

I can truly say that about every remedy suggested and recommended from the time that Bostock first wrote on the subject, 1819, had been tried, but nothing has ever given the relief and sense of comfort that this did.

One word more and I am done; the form of administration was that of the syrup—a teaspoonful every hour or two until relief.

If necessary, double the dose. The syrup, as prepared by Mr. Gardner—was the special brand, though where that is not accessible, I imagine the regular acid of the dispensatory on a lump of sugar, 3 to 5 drops, would be equally as efficacious. The mustard leaves are applied as soon as the first dose is given.

Since commencing the acid treatment, my brother, Dr. C. P. Judkins, has prescribed it in another case, that of a married lady who suffered intensely with the asthmatic symptoms, with perfect relief, that so far has been continuous, and as in my own patient, bids fair to continue so. The capsules were discontinued when commencing the use of the acid.

---

## GARDNER'S SYRUP HYDRIODIC ACID IN LUPUS, CHRONIC BRONCHITIS, AND CHRONIC MALARIAL POISONING.—"THERAPEUTIC VALUE OF GARDNER'S SYRUP OF HYDRIODIC ACID."

By W. H. BENTLEY, M. D., LL. D., COLD SPRING, WOODSTOCK P. O., KY.

(Reprinted from the *Medical Summary*, March, 1885.)

After summing up the various therapeutic advantages of iodine. and discussing the acrid and escharotic properties of it in substance, and the disadvantages of the iodides in many cases, from the objectionable character of the base in chemical combination with it, and lastly, of the advantage of Hydriodic Acid, whereby the system might be brought under the influence of iodine without most of the objectionable features spoken of, he says: "But here a new difficulty presented itself, growing out of and dependent upon the instability of the Hydriodic Acid itself, for the pure Hydriodic Acid cannot be preserved in an undeteriorated state through any considerable length. of time."

For this reason Hydriodic Acid was dissmissed from the U. S. P., in 1870. It remained however, for the chemist R. W. Gardner, of 158 William street, New York, to overcome all difficulties in regard to the unstable character of Hydriodic Acid (which he did in 1878), and to place this valuable therapeutic agent in the hands of the medical profession in an available and convenient form. This he has accomplished in the form of a permanent syrup, in which the acid is thoroughly preserved in its original purity for an indefinite period of time. I have tested its permanency in several ways, and found it stable. * * * * *

Gardner's syrup of Hydriodic Acid resembles lemon syrup in taste, and is therefore easy of administration. It should never be combined with any other drug.

Since March, 1884, I have used the syrup of Hydriodic Acid rather extensively in my practice, and consider it a prompt and efficient alterative.

I used it first in a case of lupus of two years' standing.

It was situated on the anterior aspect of the left leg, midway between the knee and ankle joints, nearly circular in form and a little more than two inches in diameter.

The patient was a nervous little woman, of light complexion, thirty-two years old, and was, at the same time, suffering from both dysmenorrhœa and leucorrhœa. Besides local measures, I prescribed the internal use of the above syrup, at first in drachm doses four times daily. The doses were gradually increased to twice that amount. The improvement was immediate and rapid. I treated the case seven weeks.

At the expiration of that time, the ulcerated surface was about the size of a twenty-five cent coin, and the patient in all other respects well. She then returned to her home in Kansas, and I lost sight of the case. [I have recently, Nov. 2, 1885, received a letter from this patient, stating that she is entirely well.]

I commenced this case April 15, 1884. May 20, 1884, prescribed syrup of Hydriodic Acid for Mr. B., a well-to-do farmer, age 54, who had been suffering with a distressing cough from chronic bronchitis for the past twenty-two years, the result of a relapse from measles. During the last ten years a gradually increasing asthma had complicated the case. Most of the time he had been under the care of some physician or quack.

The Pierces, Van Meters, and other rascals of that ilk, had during the last few years, fleeced him of hundreds of dollars. All had proved unavailing; he had all the time grown gradually worse.

At my visit I regulated his bowels and put him upon syrup of Hydriodic Acid. He began to improve immediately, and by the middle of the ensuing August was apparently well, and still remains so.

July 2, 1884, J. C., applied to me for treatment. He had, for the past eight years, resided in a malarious district of Texas. During the past seven years he had been the victim of chronic intermittent fever; unless when under the influence of quinine or some other potent drug, he had one chill every day, some days two. They would cease for a few days when taking medicine, to resume again as soon as the influence of the medicine had passed away. When examined, his bowels were confined, liver torpid, and spleen greatly enlarged and much indurated. He looked bloodless, and his skin was waxy and of an ashen hue.

I went to work, regulated his bowels, stopped his chill with large doses of dextro-quinine and Hypophosphite of Soda. I then gave him a supply of syrup of Hydriodic Acid and a strong solution of quinine, ten grains to the dose.

I put him on the syrup, two teaspoonful doses three times a day for six days. On the seventh day he got three doses of quinine and no syrup. From the eighth he had his syrup as before, until the next seventh day. Then the quinine as before, thus alternating until the fifty-sixth day. Then for a month the syrup in diminishing doses till a pint was used, never going below teaspoonful doses. He got well of all his diseases, and so remains at this writing—Feb. 20, 1885, although he has been exposed to much inclement weather since. Syrup of Hydriodic Acid has in my hands proved of the greatest benefit in the scrofulous and cutaneous diseases of children; also in mercuro-syphilitic rheumatism.

---

## ACUTE PNEUMONIA.

### By W. H. BENTLEY, M. D., LL. D., Woodstock, Ky.

(Reprinted from the *Medical Summary*, January, 1888.)

November 11, 1885, called at 10 o'clock, a. m., to see J. T.; æt. 19 years; found him with badly furred tongue, pulse 150 and full, temperature 103.5°. He complained greatly of pain in right thoracic region, coughed almost incessantly, and raised a large amount of bloody sputa. Auscultation and percussion showed that the entire anterior surface of the right lung was involved. Another physician who had called to warm himself, was present. He told me unhesitatingly that the patient was bound to die.

At 12 o'clock, noon, I administered a dessertspoonful of syrup of Hydriodic Acid, well mixed with 2 f. ℥ of water. I repeated the dose at 1 and 3 o'clock p. m., directing a similar dose every three hours during my absence.

I returned next day at noon. The tongue had greatly cleared of its furred appearance. The pulse had lost its rigid feel, and beat softly at 100. I did not take the temperature. The cough was not so harassing, and the sputum was rust-colored. Complained of little pain.

Continued medicine at intervals of four hours. Saw him 14th at 3 o'clock p. m.; all the symptoms had improved, but there was marked exacerbation of fever at night. Directed medicine continued at intervals of four hours, each dose followed in two hours by 5 grs. sulphate quinine in absence of fever.

I did not see the case again, but the patient made a rapid and complete recovery.

R. W. Gardner, of New York, the originator of this invaluable preparation, cautions against compounding the syrup of Hydriodic Acid with other drugs; but I have given many other preparations in usual doses from one and a half to two hours after the syrup, and with the happiest results, and I state this fact here for the benefit of other physicians wishing to use this syrup.

I have used the syrup of Hydriodic Acid in twenty-three cases of acute pneumonia, and always with good results. I have not the space to detail the cases.

In remittent and intermittent fevers, given in dessertspoonful doses every four hours, and followed two hours later by full doses of quinine, I have had unvarying success, and I have pursued this treatment in a number of cases.

In acute rheumatism I have never found any other drug its equal.

I kept notes of nineteen cases of acute rheumatism, treated with syrup of Hydriodic Acid—all made rapid recoveries.

One day I was sent for to see a case, supposed to be acute rheumatism. I was ill and confined to my room; I gave the messenger one pound syrup Hydriodic Acid. In a few days he returned, saying that the patient was no better. I went with him, and found that my patient had gout.

I have tried this preparation in about four cases of gout. The results have not been satisfactory.

In both acute and chronic bronchitis I consider the syrup of Hydriodic Acid of the greatest value. It is likewise of the greatest value in convalescence from measles, pneumonia and bronchitis.

It is never necessary in the administration of this remedy to wait for a fever to subside. I have thoroughly tested it in this respect.

I give the following case for what it is worth:

Capt. A., who had been a widower, and recently married to a blooming young lady of twenty, came to me in great consternation. He lived in another county, some thirty miles distant, but he brought his once lovely wife, lovely alas, no longer, for an inveterate psoriasis had seized her entire person, except the scalp, and Job himself could not have presented a more loathsome appearance. To make bad worse, several physicians had failed in the last year.

I prescribed iodide and carb. potash, Fowler's sol. arsenic and fl. ext. berberis aquifolium internally; externally, a mild ointment of oleate mercury.

He was back in a month—case no better. I then prescribed Donovan's sol. ars. internally, chrysophanic acid ointment externally; still it was "no go." He reappeared. I then prescribed syrup Hydriodic Acid, one pound.

Sig. A dessertspoonful before each meal and at bedtime; locally, a mild oleate of zinc ointment.

This did the work, leaving the skin in a perfectly natural condition.

# SYRUP HYDRIODIC ACID IN SMALL-POX.

### BY W. H. BENTLEY, M. D., LL. D., WOODSTOCK, KY.

(Reprinted from the *Medical Summary*, June, 1891.)

Prior to the war of the rebellion my experience in treating small-pox had been comparatively limited. Many of my cases were treated in a hospital in which I was interne. I was then young, and, like many young men thus situated, I inclined to shift the responsibility to the shoulders of my superiors, and to let them do most of the thinking, if, indeed, any thinking was done.

During most of the war my location and itinerant practice, in a city at all times the headquarters of an army of one or the other of the belligerants, brought me each winter into immediate contact with many cases of this loathsome disease.

The responsibility was my own, and if any thinking was done I had to do it. The text books to which I then had access recommended cold food and drinks. I soon become to distrust and then to abandon this course of practice. With the exception of an occasional cathartic, or a restrainant of diarrhœa, I gave luke-warm infusions of rattle-weed (cimicifuga, or macrotys racemosa) and mountain dittany (cunilla mariana). This course was followed in the earlier stages, and indeed, until the complete establishment of the postular period.

I observed that after this period most of the mortality in my cases occurred. I then, as I do yet, ascribe the fatality at this and subsequent periods of the disease to the absorption of pus.

I sought to remedy this by giving alteratives, mostly the iodide of potash. This was the only iodide then and there attainable.

I found this often entirely rejected by the stomach, so that its discontinuance was necessary. Among this class of patients (those who could not tolerate the iodide of potash) were nearly all my fatal cases.

Since the close of the war there have been many outbreaks of small-pox in sections where my services were sought, for many physicians, through fear or from other causes, decline to treat the disease altogether.

I have frequently gone to a small-pox stricken section fifteen and even twenty-five miles distant, and remained until by vaccination and other means the further spread of the disease was fully controlled.

I continued the use of iodides—mostly the iodide of sodium, as being the best borne—after the close of the war until 1880.

I treated no case of small-pox from 1880 until December 12, 1890. Through the remaining part of that month I had in charge, all told, thirty-one cases. These cases were all in one neighborhood and about twenty miles distant, most of them, at least, in an adjoining county. Most of the cases were comparatively mild, there being three of them of the confluent variety.

From the commencement of my use of the syrup of Hydriodic Acid, which I think was in 1884, I had thought of it in the suppurative and subsequent stages of small-pox. Its acceptability to the most delicate stomach, together with its superior alterative qualities, pointed to it as the remedy.

The evening of my arrival at the stricken village I visited the druggist to induce him to order the above-named syrup. He was an old friend and had been induced by my earliest published articles on syrup of Hydriodic Acid to give it a trial, he being also a practicing physician.

He had used it largely and in different diseases, and always, he thought, with marked benefit. I found him with a large stock of Gardner's syrup on hand. I prescribed it in the suppurative and subsequent stages up to the complete desquamation in nearly all the cases, I thought, with the happiest results. None of the cases lingered or made tardy recoveries. All got well. Experience has given me so much confidence in this course of treatment that I do not hesitate to lay it before the profession.

# SYRUP OF HYDRIODIC ACID—HOW AND WHEN TO USE IT.

### By HENRY M. FIELD, M. D.,

Professor of Therapeutics, Dartmouth Medical College, Etc.

(Reprinted from the *New England Medical Monthly*, October, 1890.)

Hydriodic Acid is a compound which in chemical symbol is indicated by the formula HI and in chemical composition consists almost entirely of iodine. This paradox of constitution, pertains to the fact that the equivalent of iodine is 127, the equivalent of hydrogen less than 1; hence a little over 99 p. c. of Hydriodic Acid is iodine. The syrup of this acid, the only pharmaceutical form in which it is used, was somewhat in use prior to 1870; but in that year was stricken from the U. S. P. on account of the uneven and imperfect methods by which it was prepared, and also its frequent instability. For several years thereafter it remained unemployed and indeed had become nearly obsolete, when, through the successful efforts of a New York chemist, it was introduced to the medical profession, being received into the general favor which it has since enjoyed. And, indeed, it was no small service which R. W. Gardner thereby rendered to practical therapeutics; the syrup of Hydriodic Acid as prepared by his method, and restored to pharmacy by his enterprise, has held its ground ever since such introduction, being of uniform strength, of stable constitution,—at least when the necessary conditions of its preservation are met,—and of agreeable taste.

The original gift and service of Mr. Gardner should always be kept in mind and receive due and grateful recognition on all proper occasions. No less than this the writer feels bound to say; and to add that there must be many physicians and druggists throughout the country, who, like himself, will always hold in pleasant memory an interview or communication of years ago, in which the information sought was freely and effectively afforded; and in a way, also, which bespoke the gentleman as well as practical scientist.

A magistral syrup of Hydriodic Acid is estimated to represent 6½ grains of iodine in each ounce, is of the consistence of lemon syrup, of agreeable sub-acid taste, of pale straw color and must be absolutely free from insoluble particles. Moreover, it may be regarded a stable compound, so long as essential conditions, both as to its keeping and use, are intelligently observed. It must not be exposed to a strong light, or left long exposed to the air; avoidance of either extreme of temperature is equally imperative. Approach to either 32° or 100° Fahr., not alone endangers the loss of medicinal properties, but makes liable a change in chemical construction, through which a positively deleterious action may result.

As already said, a good specimen of the syrup will be of a fixed, uniform color and will present translucency,—be absolutely free from insoluble particles,—and this, whether held in suspension or precipitated. A faulty preparation,—faulty at first because not made right, or afterwards because not kept as it should be,—will most often present departure from the standard in two corresponding particulars: will be *reddish or reddish-brown in color*, and to use a common word will be *turbid*. Such specimen cannot fail alone to exert the properties for which the remedy is prescribed; there is danger lest it further exert the properties of an irritant and toxic. A syrup presenting signs of reddish color and turbidity, also presents evidence of chemical decomposition, and among the products of decomposition, iodine in precipitated form.

**The Dispensing, Care and Preservation, Ingestion, Etc., of Hydriodic Acid.**—However it may be with his usual prescriptions, the physician should always give attention to the source from which this remedy is procured. It may be just that pharmacist, who has not the skill to make the preparation himself, who will often prove ignorant or indifferent as to the honesty or skill of the manufacturer from whom he buys.

Again, should the essential, initial care have been properly exercised, it is equally imperative that, the medicine once procured, a complete and intelligent understanding should exist between physician and patient, as to the treatment it shall receive, while in the hands of the latter, with purpose to ensure its continued integrity. A lack of proper attention given to the points thus made, (and to another soon to be presented, and which, if possible, is of greater moment), is chiefly responsible for partial result, positive failure, in the use of the syrup, and, too often, for unmistakable injury attending upon its use.

The *ingestion* of the remedy demands the strict attention of the prescriber; and in this particular, with the many results involved, the latter is alone responsible, as, upon details just presented, he shares responsibility, in varying degree, with the druggist. But, above all, it is a determination of *the hour with reference to eating*, when the medicine shall be taken, which is of importance, *of capital importance*; and, still here again, error, ignorance, indifference will not alone bring failure in medication, but, often, deleterious results also.

Now unless the writer is strangely misinformed, the standard books and teachers seldom give emphasis to this capital condition, as we conceive it to be, in the use of the remedy; too often, pass it by without notice. Many medicines can afford such slight and dismissal; syrup of Hydriodic Acid cannot afford it. In all that directly concerns the ingestion of this remedy, there must be conscientious instruction on the part of the physician, intelligent co-operation between the physician and patient, strict obedience of the latter to the former, or the medicine had much better never been prescribed.

Just here, and as pertinent to the immediate subject, a somewhat personal remark may be excused; first, in the writer's capacity as a writer, again in his capacity as a practitioner. As said heretofore, if he is informed upon the subject of present consideration, if his estimate of a material which has been an object of use, study, and instruction on his part for many years, is correct, we have now reached that stage of the discussion which, with purpose of all possible brevity, demands in its treatment a concession of whatever space may be required, even although as compensation, some other departments are passed rapidly and curtly in review.

As a practitioner, he is free to confess that, in early experience with the remedy, it was prescribed for some time and with repetitions before it began to be realized that there had been wrong, misconception, neglect, upon a condition more essential to the success of the remedy and the help of the patient than any other, except the remedy's initial and continuous integrity. And this condition, which concerns the hour of the day, because of the implied status of the patient's stomach, imperatively governing the exhibition of Hydriodic Acid, was first taught, not by the consultant, by standard books of reference, but by the complaints rendered by the stomachs of those under treatment. After a certain number had reported disturbances occasioned by the remedy, gastric distress, etc.; after the remedy in consequence, had been more than once suspended, condemned, abandoned, the secret of disappointment and disaster was revealed.

A universal rule in medication, seldom as such is met with, is a measure of actual help to the practitioner, who rightly apprehends it; to the specialists in therapeutics, it affords a satisfaction which may partly come from the offset it suggests to conditions continually reminding him how far removed from an exact art is the art to which he is devoted. That universal laws exist is sure, as sure as that these laws are very few. When a law that is really absolute and without exception presents, particularly if it concers practical therapeutics, it is certain to have a value and authority which we cannot well disregard. It is a common rule, and yet of frequent exception, a rule which is every day recognized and acted upon, that remedies are best ingested while there is food in the stomach, i. e., during the meal or soon after.*

On the other hand it is a *universal law*, if we mistake not, and one of opposite direction, which governs the exhibition of the medicine of present study, viz., *the syrup of Hydriodic Acid must always be presented to an empty stomach*; or as we express the condition to the patient; repeating the medicine two or three times each day, you should always take it *a half hour*, as nearly as possible, *before each meal*. We insist that this law is universal, as so established by repeated clinical evidence through the years; evidence which was personal with ourselves and that which has been communicated by other observers.

The principles, physiological and chemical, both, on which such regulation rests, can only require assertion: Hydriodic Acid, in whatever medicinal form, is an agent of frail chemical constitution: (and this fraility, which is inevitable, which pertains to the chemical nature of the body,—before remarked of it as a pharmaceutical preparation—follows it from the shop of the chemist to the closet and stomach of the patient.) Easily decomposed, on exposure to any chemical disturbance, *it must always enter a stomach which is empty of food and which is, therefore, of neutral reaction.* If the stomach receiving it be occupied with food and the digestive process, the remedy promptly ceases to be a remedy, assumes a modified form of analogy to the discolored, turbid, pharmaceutical preparation, of which we have taken previous note, becomes a local irritant and if it be absorbed, a toxic also; but with this difference, that a chemical disintergration, which occurs in the bottle (before ingestion of the remedy,) is more innocent for the patient than that taking place in the stomach.†

In conclusion, we state our belief, that a neglect to recognize and obey this law which should govern the administration of Hydriodic Acid is the most frequent and prolific cause of negative result, disappointment, disastrous results in its use.

Let it be objected that the principles concerned with the ingestion of such a remedy are obvious, are such as to justify the slight or omission experienced at the hands of many teachers and hardly to excuse the space at present devoted to their illustration, and that it may safely be left to the rational deduction, *a priori* observation of the physician. This might all be, were the medical profession, generally, a body of reasoning, observing, thinking men (and the author would enter a prompt *caveat* and disclaimer of odium conveyed in this remark, having confessed, for himself, that it was through *a posteriori* evidence, as afforded by his patient's stomachs when maltreated, that he first learned a correct practice, based upon the *universal law* enunciated.)

But all physicians have not been set right through such observation, even. In a word then, the pharmacist has learned during recent years, how to prepare and dispense the remedy; it is presumably trustworthy and efficient as it comes to us from his hands. But, before such remedy can accomplish all of which it is capable and possess the uniform, universal confidence of the profession, the physician must learn how to use it.

---

*It is, practically, a universal rule that *iron as a hæmatinic* should thus be taken; the physiology and therapeutics of the remedy are perhaps equally involved in obedience to such rule. I believe that there is but one morbid state, presenting exception to an otherwise universal law, that *arsenic* taken in course, must be received with the food.

Fonssagrieves, the ingenious author of many valuable works on practical therapeutics, strangely enough seldom given [or given but in small part] to the English reader, remarks of cathartic medication chiefly as concerns the ingestion of the aperient or laxative, that the best results in many ways, are secured by taking such remedy at meal-time *naively adding*, "*It is the English method and it is good*," intimating thereby that the French have not, as yet, learned the better way.

I am sure that one who should practice along this line, having previously practiced indifferently or otherwise, will be gratified at the modified results which will appear in his practice; and none the less there is the not infrequent occasion where it is equally important for the cathartic material to be received by an empty stomach.

†It may become exceptionally, *an essential and an active toxic. The iodates* are essentially toxic salts, thereby presenting a marked contrast with the iodides. Now if iodine be precipitated in the stomach, in a form of a minutest subdivision, at a time when the chemico-vital energies of digestion are in full operation, it may well be that conditions shall obtain calculated to invite transformation into an iodate. Against such peril it would seem that no assurance can be given, however improbable its occurrence may be, however infrequent.

\

47

That there is frequent difficulty in directing a course of Hydriodic Acid and securing its regular, repetitive ingestion at the right hour of the day, the physician cannot have failed to recognize who has had somewhat of experience in this way. It is not every patient who can so command his time as to take his medicine t. i. d., and always considerably before sitting down to table; and others, who might do this, and who remember to take their medicine at meal time, will not long remember to receive it, regularly, *at quite an interval before the meal.*

For a disability, often, in the writer's experience, is an object of respect, there is no help except as it may come from an intelligible representation to an intelligent patient. Of one thing I am sure, from long observation; the conference between doctor and patient on this point must always close with the ultimatum: *the remedy must be taken on an empty stomach or it must not be taken at all!* (and there are worthy and intelligent patients who are made all the better for the discovery, by indirection now and then, that their physician does not prescribe primarily for their convenience, but for a purpose quite different). And still, exceptionally, if the dose had been forgotten for the occasion or unavoidably delayed, it may be taken, even so near the approaching meal as by fifteen to ten minutes. If the proper relations exist between doctor and patient, the course of medication, efficiency of the medicine, will not be allowed to suffer prejudice through the neglect of minor instruction and concession like this.*

**Physiology of Hydriodic Acid.**—So true is it of the more intelligent, scientific study of medical materials which prevails in recent years, that the comprehension of the physiological functions and impression of an important drug is an essential substructure on which to erect in the more practical, clinical realm, that the physiology of a drug may even suggest certain of the more important of its applications in medication. That such is the fact in the present instance will soon appear.

But it will be consistent with the practical purpose of this paper to emphasize but one phenomenon in the physiological action of Hydriodic Acid; and such as is, by necessity, chiefly negative and made apparent by way of contrast. The various iodides, from the inorganic to the organic, are characterized by two prominent conditions of physiological impression; viz., an action which is apt to be unduly emphatic, however moderate may be the dose and brief the time of medication, occasioning a functional disturbance which often steadily increases with each repetition of the remedy; and again the modification wrought by idiosyncrasy, the introduction of complications, perversions, incapable of anticipation or prevention, and which is an extreme development, constitute the substitution of a syndroma of toxic impressions for physiological actions; although the limit of medicinal dosing has not been exceeded. Probably no other familiar remedy is so apt to produce such confusion, bringing perplexity and alarm to the inexperienced physician, and distress to the patient, as a simple, generally harmless inorganic iodide, under circumstances of pronounced perversion, as effected by some hidden, unsuspected force in the individual constitution. A drug

*Corresponding to the law, which we have sought to establish and illustrate, that the syrup of Hydriodic Acid should always be ingested by an empty stomach, is the very general antithetical law *that all other derivatives of iodine and the metalloid itself are best received by the stomach during or immediately after the repast.* This rule in medication applies to the inorganic iodides, the mineral iodides, the organic iodides; but has especial pertinency and force with the first-named class, given, as the inorganic iodides generally are, continuously and with purpose of alterative or of tonic-alterative impression. It is essential, alike to a mild physiological action and to the procurement of the surest and best medicinal action, that they not only should be received with the food, but, if we may not say digested with the food, at least absorbed and assimilated with it. The superior therapeutic force and efficacy of the remedy, thus appropriated to the wants of the system, has been shown to be procured through the operation of several distinct physiological principles: (which we cannot give here) as by the experimental studies of Duroy, et cet. We do not forget that *the iodides are not the subject* of our discussion; but the present note has the interest of antithesis, and it is believed may serve, although by the very contrast presented, still farther to illuminate a point which it is especially desired to enforce.

Even the massive doses, in free dilution, of the neurologists, one drachm or less of sodic or potassic iodide, are sometimes comfortably received by a stomach occupied with food; and I have the strong impression that my friend, Dr. Seguin, prefers such status for this medication.

which does more mischief physiologically, than it seems to do good (therapeutically), must be discontinued; and such problems or one of like element, are too often confronted in iodide medication.

And occasionally a dilemma like the following presents: The medicinal service of a derivative of iodine is found to be beneficent and essential; substitution of a remedy from some other chemical class will avail nothing—the patient, by turns, takes up and lays down again his sodic iodide: has recourse to other iodides, later to that of starch, again to the smallest (rational) doses of the offending drug—and still the physiological penalty follows him, hardly ever abating in degree. A degree is finally reached which is beyond endurance.

Now it may be doubted, with sole exception of Hydriodic Acid, if there is any derivative of iodine, of assured medicinal power, the physiological power of which is so little pronounced as frequently not to be apparent. The remark has been made already that its influence in the latter province was chiefly made evident by contrast; repeatedly, it is not declared at all, under circumstances of skilled medication, though the material be long used and often repeated. It would even seem that upon the stomach the alimentary canal and their functions, as well as elsewhere, and that upon various secretions the impression of Hydriodic Acid is as kindly, as little given to any disturbance as is its first impression on gustatory nerves and the secretions of the mouth.

Indeed this apparent absence of action, the contrast presented with what is sure to be observed in the operation of all other iodic preparations, in one degree or another, has led physicians to question the existence of medicinal properties in Hydriodic Acid; and such skepticism was quite prevalent at one time.

But the further we advance in the department of physiology in therapeutics, the more familiar we become with the physiology of drug action; the more evidence do we receive of the substantial truth of two general principles, viz., and firstly, action is not necessarily displayed in, and limited to reaction, irritation, disturbance; secondly, there are valuable and potent drugs, the physiological action of which, when they are skillfully exhibited, is alone kindly, consistent with and helpful to the purpose sought and procured in their therapeutic action. Under such circumstances the practitioner who looks for reaction, irritation, as constituting the sole evidence of impression in the physiological realm, will be disposed to deny the reality of such action altogether; and perhaps reach a further conclusion that, therefore, therapeutic action does not exist, that the remedy in review is inert and without value.*

**Therapeutics of Hydriodic Acid.**—Two "indications" present a claim for brevity in this our closing section. There would seem to be propriety in the generic presentation alone of the chief therapeutic applications of the remedy, such treatment can be dismissed in few words and a treatment otherwise, by clinical reports, is less suitable to a paper of scope like this. Again, no other opportunity will appear for us to pay respect to a previous promise of brevity at some point, as offset for the space in the pages of the journal which were so freely appropriated.

First.—The use of Hydriodic Acid (with very rare exception) wholly avoids the variously exerted irritative effects of the other iodics; and which, if they are less serious, when confronted with that grosser development of like irritation, wherein a toxic action has absolutely taken the place of a physiological, are still scarcely of less concern to the practitioner because of their much more frequent occurrence. Again, its pharmaceutical preparation offers a substitute for remedies more or less unpalatable (throughout the entire class) to the young subject, the patient with delicate stomach, and with whomever the palate may also demand respect.

Second.—As affording a substantial, often a complete relief to such patients as suffer what the writer has, many times, termed *the iodide of potassium punishment;*

---

*Sulfonal,* as treated by the writer in a portion of his paper published in the July issue of the *New England Medical Monthly* affords so apposite an illustration of the main points at issue, that he would apologize for thus quoting himself.

but with whom, arrest of medication, or a material substitution cannot be considered. These *idiosyncrasic sports* of pre-eminently, the organic salts are so extravagant, preposterous and so varied in form, that their study and report has created quite a department of itself in the literature of therapeutics; but the more striking cases, presented in the pages of Lewis, Jonathan Hutchinson, etc., might many times be offset by a record of the experience of many an observant practitioner who seldom or never contributes material to the reading medical public. But *"verbum satis;"* suggestion and experience of others must further develop in this province of exceptional moment but which we dismiss without further words.

Third.—For the less precipitate cases; cases which plainly indicate recourse to iodics but permit a choice in measures and abundant time in their application. The *more chronic conditions of asthma* may be cited prominently; emphatically whenever the iodides are not kindly received. Many conditions of *bronchial or pulmonary catarrh* show most gratifying treatment under Hydriodic Acid treatment. *Chronic accumulations of serous fluid* also demand mention in this brief review.

---

# SYRUP HYDRIODIC ACID IN THE TREATMENT OF PLEURISY.

## By LEWIS G. PEDIGO, M. D., of Roanoke, Va.

One of the most important uses of Hydriodic Acid has not received the attention its importance would seem to demand. I refer to its use in the treatment of chronic pleurisy, and its controlling the after effects of certain kinds of acute pleurisy. The two types of this disease of which I wish to speak more particularly in the present connection are:

First.—Pleurisy with slight adhesive exudation.

Second.—Pleurisy with extensive serous effusion.

I believe it safe to say that Dr. J. B. Leaming has finally succeeded in convincing the profession that a large majority of the cases of phthisis have their origin in the so-called dry pleurisy.

It is a very insidious and a very prevalent disease. Almost every autopsy within the recollection of any medical man, performed upon a subject of over thirty years of age, has revealed pleural adhesions of variable extent.

In a large proportion of these cases, pleurisy was never discovered during life. A great deal of the chronic bronchitis of which we hear so much, is really chronic adhesive pleurisy with secondary envolvement of the bronchial tubes.

This type of pleurisy, then, is of the first importance.

Firstly.—Because it is exceedingly prevalent.

Secondly.—Because it is easily overlooked in the first developments, and

Finally.—Because it is usually the initial and only curable stage of pulmonary consumption.

Given a case which has been recognized before it has gone too far for anything but palliative treatment, the urgent question is—what shall we do to arrest the morbid process in time to save the patient's life?

I feel that I can speak with something like confidence if not authority, on the subject.

Twelve months ago I had a rather severe sub-acute attack of this nature in my own person. Whatever harm it may have done, it served the good purpose of calling my attention to the chronic process which I have reason to believe had been going on insidiously for some time.

In February, '89, I was examined by eminent authorities in New York, placed under treatment, with the suggestion that I spend my future winters in a dry southern climate. This suggestion I fully intended to accept, but after following the treatment closely until July, I returned to the city for a second examination.

The distinguished medical man who had been so positive in his advice, reconsidered it, and told me that the results of treatment had so far surpassed his expectation, and that I was so nearly recovered that I might remain in my present location. A few days ago I was examined by a very careful man for admission into an insurance order; I gave him this history and mapped out for him the locality of the old trouble. He declared after thorough physical examination that he could discover no local evidence of adhesion, or any other morbid condition whatever.

Of course, other measures were not neglected, but the one essential feature of treatment which was followed and depended upon, from first to last, was the use of Gardner's syrup of Hydriodic Acid. I had every opportunity to observe effects in detail, such opportunity as can only be found in this otherwise undesirable combination of doctor and patient in one person.

And I say now deliberately, that if I were compelled to go through such a siege and were allowed only one measure of treatment, I should select the systematic use of Hydriodic Acid to be that one measure.

Without going into tedious details, I wish to mention one cardinal point. In my own case, as in many others (may I say a majority?), this tendency to pleurisy is associated with a tendency to the development of muscular rheumatism and finds its exciting cause in the peculiarities of a "rheumatic climate." Bring together, then, a "bilious rheumatic diathesis" and a climate of this character and the chances are largely in favor of pleurisy as a result. Of course, nothing can be done for the climate, but to move out of it, but we can do the next best thing, we can remove the predisposing cause. After years of patient research and experience, I find nothing which will compass that desirable object with such certainty and dispatch as the continuous use of Hydriodic Acid in moderate doses.

My patients frequently express their surprise at what they regard as the "incidental" relief to the rheumatic symptoms when the Hydriodic Acid is used.

This remedy gives us all the specific effects of iodine in this connection, and the stomach escapes the usual damage, a point of incalculable value in these cases.

In the treatment of pleurisy with abundant serous effusion, the great problem is to get rid of the effusion and to prevent its re-accumulation.

As a result of very positive clinical experience in a very large number of cases in the last twelve months, my routine practice is to perform paracentesis and give a course of Hydriodic Acid as after treatment.

In fact, if the operation is not too urgently indicated, I usually begin the use of the acid in advance, so as to have the patient's system somewhat under its influence when the operation is done. Under this plan of treatment I have never had to tap a second time but once, and never a third time in a single instance. Of course I am not so extravagant as to say that this would be the uniform result; but I do say that the treatment here outlined has produced in my hands by far the most satisfactory effects I have ever secured in "pleurisy with effusion."

Not only does re-accumulation seem to be prevented, but the temperature is controlled, and I do not find evidence of degeneration of the remnant of effusion—an occurrence which has always been one of the serious dangers of the operative treatment in such cases.

# GARDNER'S SYRUP OF HYDRIODIC ACID IN THE TREATMENT OF EXOPHTHALMIC GOITRE.

## By J. B. CARVER, M. D., Fort Scott, Kansas.

(Reprinted from the *Kansas Medical Catalogue*, October, 1890.)

Up to six years ago, all my efforts to treat this affection successfully had been useless. After a more or less prolonged trial, and various changes of medicine, the patient would gradually disappear, to my great relief.

It was about this time that I came across Hamilton's article on this disease and his recommendation of this remedy, and it so happened that a case soon presented itself. The lady had suffered three years; had tried all manner of treatment, change of climate, etc. The heart's action was so tumultuous that the entire body vibrated. She could not stand still, and of late had been unable to sleep, and it was on this mainly that she sought relief.

I persuaded her finally to try the syrup, securing a promise that she must take at least two bottles before she discarded it as worthless.

No other medicine was given except a few Dover's powders. No noticeable relief took place until after she had taken fully two-thirds of a bottle (except that she herself expressed herself better), when an almost constant uterine hemorrhage began to cease, and it was also noticed that she was stronger. The pulse could be counted at 140. From this on improvement became rapid, and by the time she had taken the second bottle pulse had fallen to 100.

She had gained in strenght and the goitre had shrunken one-half its former size, and the protrusion of the eyeball seemed less. She soon after left for home and up to a year ago had remained well.

It was either that or the following summer that Mrs. W. L. came under observation for the same disease. She had been, however, but a short time affected. She began to improve and recover by using the syrup. This summer she returned. She had waited a month, at least, before she came to me, suffering from diarrhœa and indigestion, and she could not use the syrup on that account.

For six weeks she was treated by various remedies, but galvanism of the pneumogastric was the only remedy of any effect, applied after the method advised by Barthalow—the positive under the ear and the negative at the epigastric. A five minutes' sitting would control the diarrhœa at once.

It was applied to the tumor. For a time it seemed that a cure would be effected. She became stronger, but after a time it became necessary to increase the number of cells in strength from four to as high as twenty milliamperes, without any appreciable improvement, and the treatment was dropped and replaced by the syrup spoken of. During the treatment by galvanism there had been an improvement in her digestion, and the diarrhœa totally arrested. In fact, the current unquestionably benefited her very much. Anyway, she was now able to retain the syrup, and in an incredibly short space of time her general health had rapidly improved, she gained in flesh-weight, her pulse fell to 110.

She has now taken the syrup three weeks. The value of the Hydriodic Acid as an alterative is, I believe, generally conceded, but its special value in this disease is not so well understood.

It is of interest to know why iodine in this form is so much more effective, as there is no question about its value over and above all other forms of iodine.

Two years ago we took occasion to test the remedy in a case of asthma, due, largely to fatty heart. At the first trial it seemed to be of decided benefit, but at the usual fall relapse no possible good could be noticed.

It is of decided value in children of a strumous diathesis, enlarged lymphatic glands, etc.

One great trouble is to obtain a reliable article of the syrup, and our experience is that R. W. Gardner's is the only reliable article in the market that will never fail, if fresh when bought. The syrup should be clear, and if it be of a brownish color it is unfit for use.

It may be that the acid in this combination has some influence independently of the iodine. There is no question but what the results are unattainable by any other combination of iodine.

---

## GARDNER'S SYRUP OF HYDRIODIC ACID IN CROUP.

### By J. STINSON HARRISON, M. D., WASHINGTON, D. C.

(Reprinted from the *Medical Mirror*, August, 1891.)

**Croup.**—I wish to make a statement in regard to the use of syrup of Hydriodic Acid (Gardner) in the treatment of croup.

A short time since I was called at night to see a child two years old, who was suffering with a severe attack of spasmodic croup.

The father said that the child had been suffering all day; that he had used all the ordinary croup remedies, but with no avail, and feared that his boy would die. I plainly told him I feared he would, but that I would do all I could for him.

I immediately gave him a small teaspoonful of syrup of Hydriodic Acid in a little water. At the end of the first hour, the child seemed somewhat relieved; I then repeated the dose, and at the end of the second hour, the child was decidedly improved, passed the night comfortably, and the next morning was up, playing about the room; the parents, of course, were greatly delighted, and so was the physician, as I had never used the remedy before.

A short time after this I was called to see another "croup case," child same age, treated him in the same way, hot poultice over the chest, plenty of cold water, and Gardner's syrup of Hydriodic Acid, with the same happy result.

It is now my main reliance in every case of croup, and with "la grippe" I always use it with decided advantage.

P. S.—I am not aware that anyone has used Gardner's syrup before in croup.

Subsequently, under date of Oct. 29th, the Dr. writes as follows: "I am still using Gardner's syrup of Hydriodic Acid to my entire satisfaction, in nearly all cases involving the breathing apparatus, particularly croup, laryngitis, asthma, and bronchitis; and the more I use it, the more highly I value it. It hardly ever disappoints my expectations."

Under date Nov. 2, 1891, the Dr. writes, "I am using syrup Hydriodic Acid in a case of pneumonia, with most gratifying results. I hardly know now how I should get along without it."

---

## SYPHILIS.

Dr. Richard H. Taylor, Hot Springs, Arkansas, May 19, 1889 writes: "Col. V——, a prominent citizen of Tennessee, consulted me about a very ugly sore, involving his entire nose, and which had frequently been pronounced lupus. The history of the case led me to suspect syphilis, and I resolved upon constitutional treatment. He told me that he could not take iodide potassium, as his stomach utterly repudiated it. So I suggested Gardner's syrup of Hydriodic Acid. He is now upon the third bottle and is almost well, in fact leaves for his home this week delighted with his rapid and pleasant treatment. Locally for one week, I applied the gelatine ointment of chrysarobin, which promptly relieved the intense soreness."

53

# LA GRIPPE AND SEQUELÆ.

Q. A. Bridges, M. D., Berlin Mills, N. H., Oct. 1, 1890, writes: "It may be of interest to you to know the following facts, as I noticed by your pamphlet sent me some time ago, that no other physician has had a similar experience.

Since la grippe left us last winter, I have been called to several patients who complain of having pain and a prickling sensation, not unlike that of a foot being 'asleep,' in their upper or lower extremities, or both, and growing more troublesome and unendurable from week to week.

Having tried nearly everything, and meeting only with failure, I at last hit by mere chance upon your syrup of Hydriodic Acid, and am delighted to say, it was a great success. I have given it to two patients, both of whom are over fifty years of age, in doses of twenty drops to half a drachm, before meals, and the disagreeable symptoms I have before described are all gone. I see no reason why it will not work in other cases."

# BRONCHIAL CATARRH AND CATARRHAL AFFECTIONS OF THE THROAT AND LUNGS.

F. R. Garlock, M. D., Racine, Wis., June 6, 1888, writes: "In relation to your syrup Hydriodic Acid, I can say that I have used it quite extensively in my practice. I find it to be a very superior article in cases of bronchial catarrh, and in fact in all catarrhal affections of the throat and lungs. Especially is its use very advantageous in children who are suffering from congestion of the lungs from sudden colds. I like its use much better than that of potassium iodide, as it does not nauseate the stomach, nor does it cause the other disagreeable effects of that remedy. In fact, in all cases in which iodine is indicated, the syrup of Hydriodic Acid, as prepared by you, I consider an excellent remedy.

August 8, 1889, he writes: "Since my last letter to you of the 6th of June, 1888, I have extended the use of the syrup of Hydriodic Acid (Gardner) to other complaints than those mentioned. Then I wrote to you of its application in cases of pulmonary catarrh and kindred affections. I have prescribed the syrup in catarrhal affections found in other situations; I have used the same as a constitutional remedy in vaginitis, urethritis and catarrhal affections of the intestinal tract. In these situations I have derived most decided effects.

In the chronic form of vaginitis, not of a specific nature, the remedy has the same effect to relieve the disagreeable and disgusting discharges as in any other forms of the complaint. It changes the nature of the secretion, and where it was offensive before it becomes innocuous. It acts as a disinfectant as much as many of the remedies which have been placed upon the market to be used for that purpose.

In those forms of skin diseases in which iodine is indicated it fulfills a good purpose. It is a mild alterative, and can be used in any situation in which iodine or iodide of potassium can be used, and without the disadvantages of disagreeing with an irritable stomach. I have given it to young babies who could not take the iodide of potassium.

It is almost a specific in the catarrhal affections of children; especially those which occur during the winter months. All about the great lakes of the northern United States these affections prevail to so great an extent, and the fatality from these sources is very high. The most delicate stomachs are not nauseated by the syrup.

During pregnancy, when the iodide of potassium cannot be given with safety, this syrup is most harmless. In prescribing drugs one of the most essential things is to get a pure article. Many of the so-called pure drugs are only pure in that they look clear and transparent, but chemically they are far from being pure. They have no definite standard of strength, and the physician who prescribes them does not know what effects he is to get from them till he sees its operation in the system. It is not so with this syrup of Hydriodic Acid. I have failed to find any variation in the amount of iodine which any sample contains. It is always the same and can be relied upon in every case. I have tested several samples found in the market and must say that yours stands the test best of all. A very simple test, not quantitative, is to add a little spts. nit. ether to a solution of the syrup. A reaction instantly occurs which gives a rich red appearance in the cup. Iodine is at once set free.

While this short letter will not permit me to give cases in testimony, still I would just like to mention a case or two by way of illustration.

One I will mention especially, which is as follows:

On the fourteenth day of February, 1888, I was called to see a child aged about four years, girl, who was suffering from a congestion of the lungs, with croupous respiration, with all appearances of being near its fatal termination. There was extreme dyspnœa, from the excessive secretion from the lungs. I at once began the use of the syrup in doses as follows: I made a solution of the following strength: To three ounces of the syrup I added one ounce of simple syrup, and of this mixture I gave the child a teaspoonful every two hours. I directed this till some of the symptoms of the constitutional effects should appear, which I described to the nurse. The next morning when I called I found a decided improvement in the respiration. The secretion was almost stopped and the child breathed much better. I directed a poultice of ground flax seed applied to the child's chest, and the syrup continued as before, at intervals of three hours. This was continued for the next three days, when there was no further use for the remedy. The little patient was able to sit up, and my visits were discontinued. In these cases it is a pleasure to prescribe this remedy, as it is taken without any dislike on the part of the child.

In cases of incipient consumption I do not find any remedy which is so effectual in giving relief to the excessive expectoration as this syrup of Hydriodic Acid. I give it for the first three days in doses of from one to two teaspoonfuls every two hours, together with some preparation of cod liver oil, or this remedy with maltine as found in the market. These remedies work well together, and most of the cases are benefited if not cured. In cases of consumption, scrofula and syphilis, and the chronic cases of eczema not of a specific nature, it is a most excellent remedy. In cases of eczema where the case is complicated with a syphilitic taint, this remedy is all that could be desired, if used simultaneously with the mercurial preparations usual in these complaints. It is very seldom that we find any person that cannot take the remedy. In cases in which the constitutional peculiarities were of such a nature that the patient could not take the iodide of potassium, this remedy will be found to be well borne.

I know of no better remedy in bronchitis, either chronic or acute. In rheumatism it comes as near being a specific as quinine in intermittent fever. In fact, in any case in which iodine is indicated it is the most eligible form in which to administer it. In all cases of catarrh, whether of the respiratory or of the uterine systems, I find it to be a most effectual remedy.

These remarks might be much extended, but space will not permit."

**Laryngitis (Sub-Acute).**—Dr. Garlock, June 5, 1891, writes: "I have of late been using your syrup of Hydriodic Acid for sub-acute laryngitis with good results. It is far superior to the old-fashioned preparation of chlorate of potash and tincture of the chloride of iron which is a standard remedy for that disease.

It is superior in almost every way, and especially it does not injure the teeth. It can be used for all the complaints of childhood, where the old remedies would fail from their acridity.

There are a good many imitations of the syrup placed upon the market, and many are induced to try them and fail, and the acid syrup is condemned. I can assure you

·tha* there are none which equal that which you put up. I will use no other, as I have found by experience that they do not produce the same results, and they are all more irritating than yours."

## SYPHILIS, TUBAL DISEASE, LEUCORRHŒA AND MEMBRANOUS DYSMENORRHŒA.

### By A. ROSE, M. D., LEBANON, KY.

(Reprinted from *Medical Mirror*, July, 1892.)

I regard Gardner's syrup of Hydriodic Acid as the one preparation of all others deserving of the name "alterative," and the one the medical profession has been looking for in vain.

As a tonic stimulating alterative it stands alone, in that it is the most powerful in its effects upon glandular bodies, upon mucous surfaces and upon serous membranes that has ever been known, while it is non-toxic, non-irritant and an agreeable, tolerant medicine.

Iodide of potassium, syrup of iodide of iron, or any other form of iodine compound, in comparison with this particular preparation, is not to be even remotely considered.

I have used it in syphilis, where anæmia was marked, when neither potassium iodide, syrup of iodide of iron, or mercury in any form could be tolerated for one moment; anæmia disappeared, the continuous headache instantly ceased, sore throat got well at once [with a few applications of zinc. chlorid. gr. xl aquæ, one ounce,] all glandular swellings disappeared. The gummata everywhere vanished into thin air, and the irruption was held in "statu quo" until I could give the patient a few calomel vapor baths, preceded, of course, by steam sweating.

I recommend mercurial plaster after the formula prepared for me by Seabury & Johnson [their improved formula], the same to be renewed every six days.

I use a square decimeter of the plaster directly over the spleen; this together with the syrup is sufficient to produce an agreeable cure in any given case. Only dry calomel should be used upon external sores. The acid entirely supplants the iodide of potassium and syrup of iodide of iron, both in its alterative and tonic effect.

I have tested it in all forms of syphilis—primary, secondary and tertiary. In the latter there are but few manifestations of the disease after having used the remedy. The secondary symptoms are held in abeyance until it is convenient to administer a few steam and mercury vapor baths; when by the further use of the mercurial plaster, previously mentioned, and a continued use of Gardner's syrup of Hydriodic Acid, every physician may hopefully and confidently expect the happiest results to follow at once.

This preparation is not only pleasant to the palate, but it tones up the stomach, becomes an appetizer, relieves all headache however intense, resolves glandular trouble, heals mucous and serous membranes, especially the tonsil and throat.

But there is a wide field of usefulness for this preparation that so far has been little dreamed of, viz.: In tubal disease of the ovary, rheumatism of uterus, leucorrhœa and membranous dysmenorrhœa.

My experience in gynæcology and the success following the use of the remedy proves conclusively that this preparation will excel every other preparation now known in the above-named complaints.

I unhesitatingly recommend it to my brother physicians, and can readily see its ·superiority to potassium iodide, and that it will largely supplant the latter as a means for the internal assimilation of iodine. Upon trial the reason will be apparent, and ·only equal the astonishment at the result obtained by the remedy itself. All preparations of syrup of Hydriodic Acid must be of the strength of Gardner's in order to produce the above results. This will be known by its quickly resolving itself into iodine, turning red upon exposure to heat—in which state, however, it must not be used. This is the only preparation on the market I have any faith in.

---

## EXOPHTHALMIC GOITRE.

Dr. W. B. Fletcher, Indianapolis, Ind., Oct. 23, 1893, writes: "On the 14th of August, 1893, Dr. Logan Stanley, of Fincastle, Indiana, brought to me a patient suffering from exophthalmic goitre. She was about thirty-eight years of age; the disease had existed about a year. Eyes protruding and congested—could not close the lids completely; pulse 130 to 140; breathing difficult. Seeing that Hydriodic Acid is recommended in "Wood's Hand-Book of Medicine" in the article upon exophthalmic goitre, and having your preparation at hand, I prescribed it, conjoined with rest, proper diet, etc.

The result in two months is as follows: quoting from Dr. Stanley's letter of the 22nd inst. "From August 22 to October 22, she has gained twenty-eight pounds in flesh, eats heartily and sleeps well; pulse 85 to 100, according to the exercise she takes."

In a former letter from her physician, he states that "the eyes have resumed a more natural expression, and she is feeling none of the distress or pressure that was formerly so annoying."

---

# CONSTITUTIONAL TREATMENT OF TUBERCULOSIS, STRUMOUS AND SYPHILITIC DIATHESIS.

By THOMAS H. MANLEY, M. D., NEW YORK.

(Extract from a Surgical Clinic, at Harlem Hospital, New York, October 19, 1893.)

Dr. Manley in exhibiting cases on which he had operated and on which he would soon operate, said, that it was futile and useless for one to attempt to cure many constitutional conditions which presented local lesions, without in the first place attempting to tone up the system, and after operations continuing systematic treatment until the general health was fully restored. This was particularly the case with strumous children, tuberculous adults, and a large number of those whom we suspect of suffering from secondary or tertiary manifestations of syphilis.

For this purpose many of the various alteratives might be employed with advantage. Personally he preferred a preparation known as Gardner's syrup of Hydriodic Acid, for the reason that it contains alterative and tonic properties so combined as to obviate the many objections against mercury and the potassium salts. It was the ideal way of administering iodine. It was well tolerated by the stomach, agreeable to the taste and acted with great energy. In all of those sort of bone, joint, and glandular diseases, dependent on tubercle and syphilis, his custom was to commence its use by small dosage which was steadily increased until its effects were manifest. Indeed in most cases its timely and appropriate employment would obviate the necessity of any sort of surgical interference.

# SYRUP OF HYDRIODIC ACID.

By THE LATE WILLIAM F. HUTCHINSON, M. D., PROVIDENCE, R. I.

(Reprinted from the *New England Medical Monthly*, August, 1893.)

Dr. R. W. Wilcox, of the New York Post-Graduate School, has done good service to the profession at large when he called attention to the many and certain valuable qualities of the above-named remedy. That he gave credit for the preparation of almost the only reliable form of the drug with which American physicians are acquainted, Gardner's syrup, to formulæ of Duroy and others, rather than to the well-known chemist whose study and experiment brought it where it can be safely and conveniently used, and whose name it bears, is a mark of ignorance or carelessness with which he is chiefly concerned, and a personal matter for him to settle.

To us, the fact remains that Mr. Gardner has provided a method of administering iodine that is efficient, safe and pleasant, one that pleases patients and makes long continued dosing with this powerful alterative easy and harmless.

Since 1880 I have used this syrup largely in a practice which is restricted to nervous diseases and am thus debarred from the large experience which a wider field has conferred upon many of my colleagues who speak highly of it; but in my hands it has proven of great value. When medicine must be continued indefinitely, as in some cases of sclerosis or neuritis, in small unvarying quantities, it must be in such form as will not disturb digestive organs or become physically disagreeable.

Nor must it be of cumulative nature. Thus we are prevented from availing ourselves of many valuable remedies like mercury, because of the latter tendency, and of others unpleasant to taste or smell, such as cod liver oil or bismuth, both of which assert their repulsiveness in any combination that does not destroy them.

In iodine we possess an agent endowed with several qualities of which we have constant need. It is not only alterative, but solvent and sorbefacient, and would have been in far more general use but for the fact that a large number of persons, perhaps a majority, have found that digestion was so seriously interfered with by its ingestion in the only form familiar, iodide of potash, that they would have none of it. In that form it produces a violent and disgusting coryza, with hoarseness and sore throat, sometimes so severe as to be alarming.

Some years ago, I recall ordering for a tabetic patient five grain doses of potassic iodide in syrup of sarsaparilla. The next day the man returned to me with blood-shot eyes, streaming nose and rancous voice, crying out that he had been poisoned sure, and was only withheld from swearing out a warrant for my arrest on a charge of attempted homicide, by his friend's statement that a mistake might have been made by the druggist, and he had better go slow with the doctor who was probably the only man who could correct it. To appease him, I swallowed half a dozen doses, and in a few hours was as uncomfortable as he was in the same way. That settled the matter, except that all hands, myself included, set me down for a fool who could not tell what his own medicine was going to do.

Gardner's syrup has changed all that. It is agreeable to the eyes, taste and stomach, non-irritant to mucous membranes and keeps well. It is best to keep it cool and dark, but I have a bottle in my light rooms in Providence, two years old, that has remained unchanged, and at my suggestion, Mr. Gardner has recently sent samples to a leading physician in the West Indies, who will give it a thorough test in a tropical climate.

It is too valuable a remedy to remain uncopied, but I am quite satisfied that Mr. Gardner is entitled to priority of its preparation in the form which bears his name and that his syrup is the only one of several that I have seen which remains unaltered for a length of time.

58

**Fibroid Tumor.**—Dr. H. F. Stowell, Rochester, N. Y., writes: "This tumor was a fibroid in the region of the parotid gland, of twenty years' duration. Gardner's syrup of Hydriodic Acid was used in the case.

There was a perceptible shrinkage during the first two months of treatment, after which, it remained stationary. There was however, total relief of various unpleasant sensations in the growth, which, sometimes amounted to pain.

The patient also suffered from an inveterate eczema [life-long] and this has entirely disappeared.

I have since found, that eczema is favorably influenced by the acid, and that it is very useful in syphilitic and scrofulous affections, as a substitute for potassium iodide."

---

# GRIP—CLINICAL NOTES ON THE USE OF HYDRIODIC ACID [GARDNER'S SYRUP.]

## By C. L. DODGE, M. D., KINGSTON, N. Y,

(Reprinted from the *Practitioner's Monthly*, April, 1892.)

"Case I. Private practice, W. T. T. æt. forty-five. He had an attack of the grip in December, from which he made a poor recovery. The cough persisted, his appetite returned slowly, and his general health was much below par.

Early in February, he had a second attack of the grip. This was not so severe as the first, but in his feeble condition prostrated him completely, forcing him to take his bed. His cough was very dry and "tight," causing him great pain in the left side. This was relieved by small doses of morphine and ipecac. After the cough became looser and the pain subsided, I gave him two-dram doses of Gardner's syrup Hydriodic Acid three times a day, with small doses of quinine and whiskey. He made a perfect recovery and is looking and feeling better than he has in years.

Case II. Private practice, J. C., laborer. He had had several attacks of pneumonia and has 'weak lungs.' He had a very severe attack of grip in December, from which he made a very slow recovery. I used the syrup Hydriodic Acid in the latter stages with decided benefit. He had a second attack early in March, accompanied with several severe hemorrhages from the lungs. After employing the usual remedies for the hæmoptysis and enjoining perfect rest in bed for a week, or more, I began again with syrup Hydriodic Acid. He soon began to improve, the cough gradually disappeared, and his strength slowly returned. He is now at work on a farm."

**Idiopathic Asthma.—Syphilis.—Lead Poisoning with Wrist-Drop.**—Louis Lewis, M. D., M. R. C. S., Philadelphia, late of London, writes: I think it may interest you to know that I was in the habit of prescribing your "syrup of Hydriodic Acid" frequently in my London practice, with real success, in cases of idiopathic asthma, and also in syphilis. I used to obtain it through Messrs. Allen & Hanburys, and extolled its employment in these cases, through the medium of the *British Medical Journal.* Since my settlement in this country, I have still continued to recommend it, and hold letters from medical men confirming my experience of its value. I have also found it of great value in a case of lead poisoning, with wrist-drop.

# SYPHILITIC PHTHISIS.

## By WILLIAM PORTER, M. D.

Physician to the Throat and Chest Department of the Protestant Hospital, St. Luke's; Consulting Physician to the City Hospital, St. Louis.

(Reprinted from the *New England Medical Monthly*.)

Among the many causes of chronic processes in the lung a very important one is syphilis. It is probable that many of the good results which have formerly been attributed to the use of the iodides in phthisis have been attained because the condition was syphilitic rather than tubercular.

Be that as it may, we now have abundant proof of the fact that syphilis does cause a chronic deposit in the lung which, in both its local and constitutional tendencies, may resemble, and often be mistaken for, tubercular phthisis.

In a paper read before the Missouri Medical Society, in 1877, I endeavored to show that syphilis might invade the lung in different ways. The cases reported in that paper were, so far as I can learn, the first recorded histories of syphilitic phthisis in this country, although Fournier had given his well-remembered lecture the previous year, and Goodhart's reports in London were published the same year.

In May, 1888, eleven years after, I had the pleasure of again reviewing the subject before the same association. The position was no longer a doubtful one. Many contributions had been made to the subject during a decade, and many cases recorded.

So much testimony has been offered by competent observers as to the existence of a condition which we may well call syphilitic phthisis, that I will not cite cases in affirmation, but will discuss briefly several of the manifestations of syphilis as found in the lung.

In both of the papers to which I have referred these propositions were offered:

1. From syphilis may result specific deposit or gummata in the lungs resembling the nodules formed in tubercular disease.

2. Syphilitic processes may cause arterial occlusion in the lung.

3. Syphilis may give rise to a fibrous exudation in the lung, or specific fibrous phthisis.

4. Syphilis may hasten the development of ordinary phthisis by weakening the power of resistance in a constitution in which there is a tubercular tendency.

**Pulmonary Gummata.**—In support of the first statement, in 1877 I had but the history of a single case which I recalled as almost typical, and though the final proof was wanting in this case, I felt justified at the time in citing it as a case of syphilitic deposit in the lung.

A number of cases have since come under my notice, in which the history, the associated symptoms and the result after the exhibition of specific medication left no doubt in my mind as to the nature of the invasion.

While detailed accounts of individual cases would be burdensome, I will give briefly the conclusions of a few of the many writers upon the subject.

Schnitzler [Vienna, 1880] describes infiltrations of the lung and speaks of the importance of distinguishing between tubercular and syphilitic phthisis. Goodhart, Fournier, and Virchow have done much to impress the importance of this subject, while in America valuable contributions have been made by Dr. E. T. Bruen, in *Pepper's System of Medicine*, and Dr. W. H. Porter, in the *New York Medical Journal*, August, 1885.

Gummata are not so frequently found in the lungs as in other organs of the body, and are generally associated with other local manifestations.

**Syphilitic Disease of Pulmonary Blood Vessels.**—That syphilitic processes may cause arterial occlusion in the lung is susceptible of proof, but the few cases recorded may be fairly relegated to the first or third classes, *i. e.*, to those in which gummata are found, or to those characterized by fibrous exudation. A blood vessel may be pressed upon by a syphilitic deposit, or small nodules may develop within its walls, or contraction, due to fibrous tissue, may encroach upon its caliber. The injury to the vessel is a complication, but the local condition is the gummata, or the newly-formed fibroid tissue.

**Specific Fibroid Change in the Lung.**—The third proposition, that syphilis may give rise to a fibrous exudation in the lung, is a most important one.

Many writers believe that a fibroid change, an interstitial new formation, is the characteristic pathological process in the majority of cases of pulmonary syphilis. Dr. Pancritius, a general practitioner of Berlin, published a work of 300 pages in 1881 on syphilis of the lung. While he does not claim to have found a large number of syphilitic cases that had pulmonary gummata, he has noted an interstitial pneumonia with fibrous exudation along the course of a bronchiole or pulmonary artery.

Dr. W. H. Porter, in his essay of eighteen months ago, already referred to, carefully describes new connective tissue change as "broad bands closely resembling tendon tissue, which, also, involves the vesicular walls." Oftentimes the structure between the capillaries and the air vesicles is much thickened. This necessarily renders the interchange of gases more difficult, and explains in part the dyspnœa so often attendant upon the disease when the lung is greatly involved. Sometimes fibroid thickening is found in the small bronchi, and even the vesicular spaces contain inflammatory exudation. The changes taking place in the vesicles, as found by this author, are so interesting that I will quote his record in full.

"(a) The air spaces are filled with red blood disks, leucocytes, desquamated epithelium, and fibrillated fibrin, identical with that found in the second stage of a lobar pneumonia."

"(b) Others were filled with large, round, distinctly nucleated epithelial cells, with a diameter varying from one fifteen-hundredth to one two-thousandth."

"(c) Others were filled with discolorized round cells, as in gray hepatization of lobar pneumonia."

"(d) Others contained a granular degenerating material which would not stain. The marked features of these changes was that all four conditions were irregularly intermingled as though in each air sac it ran its course independently of all the rest, going through the red and gray hepatization; at this point degeneration, rather than resolution, set in. The thickened walls prevented absorption, and the degenerating inflammatory products probably account for the copious expectoration. This process is best classed as a degenerative pneumonia and one peculiar to syphilis."

Bruen says that the interstitial new formation of which we have spoken "is often evoked by antecedent catarrhal inflammations." The smaller bronchi are narrowed, or even excluded, and new blood vessels are freely produced.

Greenfield and Goodhart believe that the vascularity and high grade organization of the new growth renders it pathologically distinct from ordinary tubercular processes.

Virchow and Green maintain that in syphilis the interstitial changes are among the first pulmonary lesions, while in phthisis the fibroid change is secondary, or, at most, simultaneous with changes in the alveoli.

Much more proof might be adduced to show the existence of a fibrous exudation in the lung due to syphilis and having distinct characteristics.

**Tubercular Phthisis in Syphilitic Subjects.**—Whatever diminishes the power of resistance to disease in the human subject is a special invitation to an invasion of phthisis. Syphilis in this way is often a forerunner of tubercular phthisis, especially if in the specific treatment due care is not taken to support the strength and aid proper assimilation. I believe that too much stress cannot be laid upon this point, for we have all of us seen instances of rapidly progressing phthisis following in the wake of syphilis, where there was no evidence of either gummata or fibroid processes, but in which were all of the symptoms of tuberculosis, even to the existence of the bacillus.

It is probable that pulmonary syphilis is sometimes inherited. The autopsies made by Balzar and Brandhomme (*American Lancet*, 1888) upon syphilitic stillborn children showed characteristic syphilitic changes. Virchow, Lebert, and Depaul have described syphilitic nodules in the lungs of children, while Dr. Furgerson (*Medical News*, 1885) reported a number of cases of phthisis in children where recovery took place after the administration of specific medication.

Pulmonary syphilis unaccompanied by lesions elsewhere is rare. Oftentimes it is associated with laryngeal complications. The pathological change may occur in any part of the lung. Schnitzler found that the middle and lower lobe were most frequently affected. Bruen found the most frequent evidence at the base, while Dr. W. H. Porter believes that the apex is generally first affected, and that the lesions diminished from apex to base. In thirteen cases, including two under care since my last paper was written (May, 1888), the lesion was found in the lower lobes in seven and the apex in four. In the other two cases the middle lobe of the right lung was involved.

**Diagnosis.**—A history of syphilis and syphilitic lesions of other organs than the lung will, of course, arouse suspicion as to the cause, but in some cases even these are absent. The co-existing complications which I have found most frequent are syphilitic laryngitis and periostitis.

The physical examination in a typical case will show a well-defined area of dullness with the respiratory murmur in other parts of the lung normal. The line of demarkation between the healthy and the diseased structures is often clearly demonstrable both by percussion and ausculation. The absence of the tubercle bacillus and improvement under syphilitic treatment are, with the evidences·before mentioned, nearly conclusive.

**Treatment.**—When a case of syphilitic phthisis is first seen there will be, generally, in consequence of the advanced stage of the disease, an immediate demand for tonics and good nutrition It is impossible to make much progress in such a case unless the funclions of assimilation and secretions are stimulated.

"The mixed treatment," combining mercury and the iodides, have been for a long time held in high esteem. I have been in the habit of ordering the biniodide of mercury ointment locally where the lesion is well defined, especially if there is much pain. The counter-irritation seems to be of value here. More recently, and where there is much debility or where the iodides cannot be borne or freely used, I have been using Hydriodic Acid with good result.· I have been led to consider it an almost necessary agent in all cases of syphilitic disease of long standing of the lung or air passages. In combination with chlorodyne (made by Squire's formula) I find Hydriodic Acid available in cases with much cough or asthma.

The great objection to Hydriodic Acid has been that it is so susceptible to change from heat and air that it is difficult to keep it of uniform strength. This objection has been overcome by Mr. R. W. Gardner, of New York, whose syrup of Hydriodic Acid is practically a permanent solution, as well as pleasant to the taste.

It must not be forgotten that in the successful treatment of syphilitic phthisis and laryngitis, not only should the patient be nouished, but such remedies selected as will act specifically and yet not interfere with assimilation.

**Fatty Degeneration of the Heart—Amyloid Liver—Obesity.**—F. A. Burrall, M. D., 48 West 17th Street, New York, June 29, 1884, writes: "I have been using your syrup of Hydriodic Acid for some time, and regard it as a valuable remedy in glandular enlargements, obesity, and fatty degeneration of the heart. It seems to me to afford an excellent method for exhibiting iodine. I saw one case of enlarged liver supposed to be amyloid, in which the gland diminished as shown by measurement while the patient was using this remedy. This may have been only a coincidence, but the fact was very apparent.

"I regard the medicine as a very valuable addition to our list of remedies."

**Capillary Bronchitis, Fibroid Tumors, Syphilis.**—James A. Williams, M. D., 164 West 34th Street, New York City October, 22,1886, writes: No doubt ere this you have forgotten all about the promise I made a year or two ago, namely, to report to you the results of two or three bottles of your syrup of Hydriodic Acid, sent to me on trial. At this late date I briefly state a few facts as follows:

Two years ago I contracted (from exposure) a severe attack of capillary bronchitis, confining me to my room most of the winter. As spring and warm weather approached, I hoped to lose my cough, which was very severe, but did not.

As I was preparing to go to the country the following summer one of your agents called with a bottle, or sample, of your syrup of Hydriodic Acid, saying you claimed for it special virtue in bronchitis. I requested a bottle or two sent to me to test in my case. It was sent. I took a few doses and went off to the country, forgetting to take the medicine with me; and, thinking the change of climate would cure me, I did not send for it. I improved, but, returning to the city in the fall, grew worse. I began to arrange for a trip south for the winter. Accidentally I came across the bottle of acid I had forgotten all about, then decided to give it the trial I had promised. I took it a few days and felt better, and stopped it, not believing it was due to the medicine. I grew worse very soon, gave it another trial, and in less than ten days I was very much improved. I again ceased taking it, and in a few days began to cough more. It is frank to say I did not have much faith in the medicine. After discontinuing it several times, growing worse each time, and improving every time I resumed its use, I was cured—not of my cough, but of my incredulity relative to its merits in my case. I soon after had such confidence in its helping me, that I gave up my trip south and worked, subjected to more or less exposure, all winter. I improved and gained in weight. I used it during the winter whenever I had a return of cough, and came out sound and well; and your acid will always have the *credit*, and *you* my sincere thanks. I should have mentioned that some time in October following you sent me a bottle to test in another case, Mrs. Dr. B., who had gone through a similar experience at the same time I had, with capillary bronchitis, and left her with a very troublesome cough. It was equally efficacious in her case.

In January last I began to prescribe it, and now regret I did not keep notes of all cases.

Miss F.—bronchitis—one year—much improved after taking it a few weeks.

In March was called to see Mrs. W., an elderly lady, about sixty-eight years of age, very feeble, with profuse bronchorrhœa, with which she had been afflicted for many years. At the time I was last called she had tubercular deposits in the apices of both lungs and so feeble she could not turn in bed. I did not believe that any medicine would be of much use to her, but concluded to try the acid. She improved, and after two months was able to go about, and as well as she had been for years, but not cured.

Mrs. N., about sixty-five, had suffered twenty-five years with asthma, from bronchitis; could not lie down when I first saw her—in six weeks so far improved that she left off treatment.

Mrs. L., aged about fifty. Bronchitis, five years; scarcely able to go up one flight of stairs; has taken it a few weeks with fine results.

After testing it in bronchitis with satisfactory results, I decided to use it in other cases.

February last Mrs. George M., aged about forty, called to consult me relative to a "fibroid tumor" of the breast about the size of an orange. It was growing, and, she said, becoming quite painful; I have known her for ten years; she was always a thin, delicate lady. I put her upon the acid treatment and local applications of tincture iodine. I soon found the tumor was being absorbed, and she growing fat. After three months' treatment she returned to her home in Connecticut, having gained twenty-five pounds, with scarcely a trace of the tumor. I directed her to keep up the treatment for a few weeks longer.

About two months ago Mr. M. S., from California, called relative to a paralytic stroke, which occurred about six months ago, affecting all the left side. He had been under treatment in hospital and elsewhere with little improvement. He was pale, thin, nervous and not able to walk alone. Suspecting the trouble to arise from syphilis (he had a chancre ten years ago), he has been taking Hydriodic Acid and twice a week electricity. He has gained fifteen pounds; comes to see me walking alone, with the aid of a cane, with a wonderful improvement in the paralysis looking and feeling like a different man.

Miss S., about twenty-five years of age, came July last with a tumor of the breast. It started to develop about five years ago, which I suspected to be adenoid. After taking the acid she improved in health and weight, but complained of its becoming quite painful, and not finding it decreasing after thirty days' treatment decided to remove it, and did so. It proved to be a cystic tumor. I mention this case as the results of the operation were a little unusual, as it was done in August. After dissecting out the tumor, with the kind assistance of my neighbors, Drs. Amway and DeWolfe, we inserted a drainage tube, then stitched and strapped up the wound. Next day I removed the tube; third day eight or ten stitches were taken out. On the sixth day it had healed perfectly, without one drop of suppuration, none present even on removing stitches, all healing by first intention. It is my belief that the previous acid treatment contributed largely to this result, and I shall in future make further trial of it previous to operating.

About three months ago Mrs. M., aged thirty-eight, called relative to tumors—one on the neck and one on the side. Acid and electricity have been the treatment, she has gained about fifteen pounds. The tumor on the neck is all absorbed; the one on the side about three-fourths. She is feeling finely and looks quite like a young miss.

That Hydriodic Acid is one of our best agents in bronchitis, proof is not wanting.

That it is very efficacious in absorbing tumors, nodes and a variety of non-malignant growths, some of which may in time become malignant, I have no doubt.

That it will add flesh and improve the general health of nearly all, if not all, is no longer a question with me.

I am now testing it in scrofula, tuberculosis, anæmia and debilitated cases, especially when I suspect inherited maladies, with very satisfactory results.

I find other makes now in the market, but have not tried them. I have thoroughly tested yours and not found it wanting. I have no time to try others. I trust you may be able to keep it up to the present standard, and if so, from its sale alone, you should never want for bread.

I find the best plan is to give a teaspoonful in an ounce of water, and in a few days increase to a teaspoonful and a half, adding a little more water as the patient may desire. This, as a rule, is, I think, quite sufficient and will improve the appetite when a larger dose will sometimes act to the contrary.

**Lumbago.**—Chas. Lengel, Kansas City, Mo., September, 1885, writes: On account of the great value of your syrup of Hydriodic Acid as a medicine, and the signal service it has rendered me, I wish to make the following statement:

I have practiced medicine about twenty-nine years. Am stout and healthy and am fifty years of age.

On the 27th of February last I contracted a severe cold. Next morning, upon getting up, was very stiff and sore. As I was preparing to leave the office, was struck with lumbago, thrown to the floor, and became entirely helpless. I sent for the best physician in my neighborhood, whose diagnosis was lumbago. I told him to give me an injection (hypodermic) of morphia and atrophia, which somewhat relieved my unbearable pain.

I was ordered lithiated hydrangea ʒ j every three hours. A few hours afterwards a second physician visited me; who prescribed cinchonia salicylate, gr. v. every three hours, and emplast sinepis to my spine; still my misery increased.

Cupping was tried, and hypodermic injections repeated twice a day. One professional brother comforted me by the opinion that "I would be laid up a month or so."

The fifth day I was taken worse, my urine being hot and of a very high color, and could only be voided with great difficulty. About noon your pamphlet was handed me. After giving it a careful reading, and not having previously heard of your preparation, I concluded at once to try it. My druggist sent me only eight ounces, as there was only one pound in the whole city. I took 3 iij every two hours all night and next day up to six P. M.

After I had taken 3 vj I felt a desire to urinate, and not having been able to move an inch twenty-four hours before, I now arose without difficulty and was very much relieved of pain.

I went again to bed and took the medicine as before. Next day (Sunday,) three P. M. I was called to see a patient. When I returned I did not again take to my bed, but sat down in my office writing editorial matter, as I am the chief editor of a newspaper. As I had but little of the syrup left, I reduced the dose to 3 ij every four hours. I took the last on Monday night and felt considerably improved. My druggist ordered more of the Acid, as I was fearful of a relapse. I was obliged to wait eight days for it. All the week I attended to my extensive practice, and wrote, every night, a few columns of editorial matter.

I hardly know how these remakable results became so quickly known, but during the next week your syrup of Hydriodic Acid could be bought by the dozen in this city.

Other physicians used it at once. I myself prescribed it, since, very often for rheumatism, asthma, and hay fever, etc., with great satisfaction in every single case of that kind.

It seemed to be my duty to send you this statement of facts to render you my hearty thanks, and to recommend it to the medical profession for further trial.

June 30, 1888, he writes: In addition to my last letter I wish to state I have since prescribed your syrup Acid Hydriodic in many cases of rheumatism, asthma, hay fever, bronchitis, and laryngitis, with excellent results. It has given me more satisfaction in these cases than any remedy I have used during my thirty years of practice.

I know I was the very first physician to use it in this city, as I could get only eight ounces of it when I first prescribed it, while it is now obtainable at every respectable drug store. The cure of lumbago (in my own case,) in three days seemed to awaken a great interest in it among our physicians. One year after my first attack of lumbago I had another spell of it, which was promptly relieved by four ounces of your syrup. There is not a day that I do not prescribe it with general satisfaction to myself and patients.

I would caution physicians to see that decomposition has not occurred, generally caused by the careless manner druggists handle it. If decomposed, I have it exchanged at once. I shall certainly continue the further use of it, and recommend it to every brother practitioner, with the assurance that he will not be disappointed in giving your syrup of Hydriodic Acid a fair and impartial trial wherever indicated.

**Asthma.**—J. W. Daniel, M. D., Houston, Texas, Jan. 16, 1886, writes: "I am just now in receipt of the fourth edition of your pamphlet, calling attention of physicians to your preparations, more especially the syrup Hydriodic Acid. Some three years since, my attention was directed to this preparation (by an article, I think, published in the *New York Medical Record* )in the treatment of asthma. I immediately ordered through the druggist, several pounds of your preparation. My mother was a chronic asthmatic; one pound of the preparation (syrup Hydriodic Acid) relieved her entirely; only at long intervals now is there any indication of return of the disease, a few doses of the syrup relieving her at once.

Mrs. P., for some years a sufferer during the autumn and winter, has entirely recovered after the use of the remedy for a short time. There has been no return of the disease with .her.

Mrs. G., and elderly lady and for many years a great sufferer from asthma, has been relieved almost entirely. In this case there may be cardiac complications; still the relief has been positive for the time being; sufficient time has not elapsed to determine the permanency of it.

I am treating acute and chronic rheumatic conditions with the preparation with marked benefits. Also in secondary and the more advanced stages of syphilis, with results highly satisfactory. I am much pleased with the preparation as made by you, and am prescribing it constantly.

My druggist has been making a syrup of Hydriodic Acid and filling my prescriptions with it, but my patients complain that it does not act like the medicine they have been taking, and that the "last" was entirely different from your article."

Under the date of July 6, 1888, Dr. Daniel writes as follows: "I have used your preparation of the syrup of Hydriodic Acid constantly and exclusively since my letter to you, in bronchial and catarrhal asthma, and consecutive conditions of syphilis, rheumatism, and in glandular enlargements (scrofulous). My success in these cases has almost been phenomenal, and I am more than gratified to be able to add my endorsement of a preparation which has given me such unvarying results."

**Chronic Rheumatism.**—S. T. Yount, M. D., Lafayette, Ind., *Medical Waif*, June, 1890, writes: "*Syrup Hydriodic Acid* has been used with the best of results in chronic rheumatism. Two cases, one of one year and another of six year's standing, were cured in a month's time by the use of this remedy. The case of six year's standing had resisted all remedies, and the patient was bedridden about half the time.

*Gardner's syrup of Hydriodic Acid* was used in tablespoonful doses every four hours, and a perfect recovery ensued. It produced no gastric irritation whatever."

**Bronchitis, Scrofula, Catarrh, Etc.**—L. S. Nicholson, M. D., Washington, D. C., Nov. 22d, 1890, writes: "The best success has attended the use in my practice of your syrup of Hydriodic Acid in bronchial disorders, scrofulous troubles, uterine catarrh, enlarged glands and chronic rheumatism. In these troubles I consider it almost a specific.

Also, happy results have been obtained from the use of Gardner's syrup of Hypophosphites of Lime, Soda, Iron and Potassium, in many of those cases of racking nervous coughs, indicative of approaching bronchial and pulmonary troubles.

So that I feel it my duty to recommend these hypophosphite syrups in every case of consumption, and especially in its incipient stage."

**Potts' Disease, Chronic Bronchitis.**—Dr. Franklin Jno. Kaufman, Syracuse. N. Y., writes: "I wish to express my high appreciation of your syrup of Hydriodic Acid. I have used it with excellent success in a very aggravated case of chronic bronchitis, after everything else failed. I consider it a most wonderful remedy. In the treatment of strumous glands, nothing equals it. I would also say that I have had remarkable success in several cases of Potts' disease of the spine, by the use of your syrup Hypophosphite of Lime in alternation with your syrup Hydriodic Acid."

**Syphilis.**—In noticing an article by Dr. Judkins in *N. Y. Medical Record*, the editor of the *Medical World* writes: "We have been prescribing this in the form of Gardner's syrup of Hydriodic Acid for the past three years, with much benefit in idiopathic asthma, and also in syphilis; in the latter diseases it acts satisfactorily when iodide potassium seems to fail."—*Medical World*, May 1885, p. 163.

**Asthma, Obscure-Abscess.**—Dr. J. C. Wilson, Morley, N. Y., under date June 26, 1885, writes: "I have used your syrup Hydriodic Acid now for some months, and have been agreeably surprised at its success in treatment of asthmatic cases. I have used it in one bad case of asthma with very flattering results. I am prescribing it now in a case of obscure abscess. The patient has been seen by one eminent diagnostician, and he as well as other physicians has been unable to locate the abscess, but from facts in the case, there is no doubt of the abscess, and that it is discharging through the lungs.

It was observed that under tonic treatment the patient was losing one pound in weight per day, until put upon syrup Hydriodic Acid. This was given in dessertspoonful doses, with the result of decreasing the loss of weight steadily."

November, 1891, the doctor writes: This patient continued to improve, the loss of weight at once began to decrease, and in the course of three or four months the patient was as well as ever."

I have treated quite a number of cases of acute inflammatory rheumatism with the syrup Hydriodic Acid, and with great good results, and good results so soon, as to surprise both myself and the patients. In one case of what I believed to be acute inflammatory rheumatism I failed completely, but after seeing the patient for many months, after partial recovery, and watching him carefully, I think the disease was simply 'obesity,' with something of a gouty nature about it."

**Chronic Trachial Trouble, Cystitis, Asthma, Croup.**—Dr. J. M. Blakesby, Germantown, Ky., Feb. 28, 1890, writes: "I have been using your syrup of Hydriodic Acid, in my own case, for a trachial affection of chronic nature, for two months, am on my last bottle, and so well in that respect I deem it unnecessary to use more, at least at present. I have used it in a case of chronic cystitis, in which much relief was experienced from pain and other symptoms; I consider it an excellent remedy in this disease.

If seems to be, in my hands, all that you claim for it in the treatment of asthma and croup."

**Typhoid Fever.**—Dr. B. F. Gardner, Atlanta, Ill., March 28 1890, writes: I have been using your preparations for some time, and could not practice without them. I am particularly attracted to syrup Hydriodic Acid. I use it in typhoid fever, or whenever I find a dry, red tongue, and always get good results. In rheumatism in children it is a specific if there is such a thing.

**Chronic Asthma, Rheumatism, Syphilis, Fibroid Tumor.**—J. Weichselbaum, M. D., Savannah, Georgia, Oct. 17, 1889, writes: I have been very much pleased with syrup of Hydriodic Acid, and have been prescribing it largely. In chronic asthma and chronic rheumatism I have received no benefit from it, but in acute cases it worked charmingly. I prescribe it in all glandular troubles, and meet with success. In chronic bronchitis in two marked cases it worked nicely; the cases were in patients over seventy years of age. I prescribe it in all cases where I want to use iodine internally.

I have a case of fibroid tumor under its use, and another with syphilitic rheumatism, in which I used it in combination with hydrarg. bin-iodide with good results.

**Exophthalmic Goitre, Rheumatic Neuritis.**—Dr. I. N. Love, St. Louis, Mo., in article on "Hot Springs," in the *Medical Mirror*, May, 1891, writes: "The eminent Dr. J. M. Kellar, known all over America, reported to me a serious case of exophthalmic goitre, treated successfully by Gardner's syrup of Hydriodic Acid.

As remarked by Dr. Kellar, 'One blue bird doesn't make a summer, but summer surely is near when blue birds appear.'

Undoubtedly the absorption of plastic matter and the reduction of an abnormal circulation is aided by the internal administration of iodine, and this ideal medicament cannot be better given, than through the medium of Gardner's syrup of Hydriodic Acid.

The writer possesses, as do many others, a marked idiosyncrasy against the iodide of potassium, and when suffering recently from a rheumatic neuritis affecting the brachial plexus superinduced by a severe cold following la grippe, he was forced to relinquish the potassium iodide altogether.

Gardner's syrup of Hydriodic Acid acted admirably and it should commend itself to the practitioners at Hot Springs."

**Chorea.**—I. N. Love, M. D., St. Louis, in the *Medical Mirror*, Feb., 1891, under the head of "Chat Concerning Children," the editor refers to the treatment of chorea, and says: "As a special builder up of the nerves, the compound syrup of the Hypophosphites is indicated.

Gardner's syrup of Hydriodic Acid has in my hands proved of great value; teaspoonful doses three times a day. This, together with an available form of iron, the old-fashioned muriated tincture of iron in ten drop doses three times a day, well diluted, to the average child is of great service."

67

**Definite Strength and Reliability.**—F. F. Dickman, M. D., Fort Worth, Kansas, *Medical Catalogue*, October, 1891, says: "Gardner's syrup of Hydriodic Acid. Too much credit cannot be given Mr. Gardner in keeping this excellent preparation up to a standard of excellence and purity found in none of the numerous imitations that are found in the shops. In fact we have found that almost invariably when failure of beneficial results are reported, that some other manufacturer's product has been dispensed.

It is unfair to blame the drug or to decry it as worthless unless a good article has been used. We know Gardner's syrup to be an excellent remedy, and when recommending the preparation we mean the original Gardner's syrup and not an imitation.

**Rheumatism, Bronchitis.**—W. T. Peyton, M. D., Louisville, Ky., March 1, 1890, writes: "I cannot find words enough to praise your syrup Hydriodic Acid. It answers every indication in acute and chronic rheumatism, bronchitis, and all the morbid conditions mentioned in your pamphlet."

**Eczema.**—F. E. Daniel, M. D., Editor *Daniel's Medical Journal*, March, 1890, writes: "Gardner's syrup of Hydriodic Acid has a wide therapeutic range, but its most brilliant powers are brought out in eczema, that protean disease which so baffles the doctor, and in scrofula."

Jas. Lewis Howe, M. D., Dean Hospital College of Medicine, Louisville, Ky., June 20, 1891, writes: "Some time ago you sent to the Hospital College of Medicine an assortment of the preparations manufactered by you, with the request, that we use them in the clinics of that institution.

Permit me to say, so far as I can say in every instance they have proven of inestimable value, and I hope that you may meet with the success that you so richly deserve."

**Enlarged Tonsils.**—Extract from an article on "Treatment of Enlarged Tonsils by Injections of Churchill's Tincture of Iodine," W. D. Blatchely, M. D., Fort Scott, Kansas. From the *Kansas Medical Catalogue*, December, 1890. "At this visit on the 12th, I injected the tonsils in both cases with Churchill's tincture of iodine. The weather becoming bad they did not return to the office any more that winter. The father reported both children improved but not well.

April 23, 1890, both the last two cases were brought to me again for treatment, and the injections were resumed at intervals of two or three days. After two weeks of treatment the girl was well, but the boy was more difficult to influence, and I put him on the use of Hydriodic Acid about the first of May, in addition to the local treatment, which was continued at intervals varying from two to five days, until May 30. I have not seen his throat since that date, but the parents report him well."

**Asthma.**—Dr. C. F. Huddleston, Troy, N. Y., writes: "In an aggravated form of asthma, accompanied with chronic bronchial inflammation and some emphysema, in which I am using it, I find it to be attended with very pleasing results. Not less satisfactory results are obtained from its use in syphilitic trouble, where it is necessary that the patient have a fair amount of iodine.

In the use of potassium iodide the stomach is very apt in a short time to become irritable, and it is then found that the syrup of Hydriodic Acid acts beautifully, and with all the results to be expected from the former remedy."

# A CASE OF REFLEX ASTHMA FROM NASAL STENOSIS.

## By CHARLES H KNIGHT, M. D., NEW YORK.

(Reprinted from the *Jouna. of the Respiratory Organs*, March, 1890).

Cases of reflex asthma, due to intra-nasal disease, have ceased to be clinical curiosities. Yet brief notes of the following case may be of interest, the asthmatic symptoms having been so persistent, the nasal lesion being so marked, and the relation of cause and effect being apparently so clear.

The patient was an unmarried woman, a brunette, twenty-three years of age, and of a decidedly nervous temperament. She was a mouth breather, owing to a large hypertrophy of the right inferior turbinated body and to the presence in the left nares of a septal ridge, extending from the floor of the nose, just within the nostril, upwards and backwards to the left middle turbinated body. Thus the left inferior meatus was nearly, and the middle meatus completely, occluded.

She came to the throat clinic of the Manhattan Eye and Ear Hospital on October 19, 1889, in the midst of a severe attack of asthma. She stated that she had been subject to the disease "as long as she could remember." She was afraid to leave the house in damp weather, could not enter a room that was being swept, and was sure to have an attack after inspiring tobacco smoke. The longest period of immunity she had known was four months, a year ago, (November to March), when she observed the strictest precautions as regards exposure to known exciting causes, and at the same time made free use of cocaine as a nasal spray.

Her general health was much impaired, she lost flesh, and became unfitted for any occupation whatever.

She was given a nasal wash of Dobell's solution, and was directed to take a teaspoonful of syrup of Acid Hydriodic (Gardner's), every four hours.

Ten days later I removed the ridge from the septum with the nasal saw, making a free passage for air through the left nostril. On her next visit she said she felt much better, and her whole appearance indicated decided improvement. Her breathing, which had been constantly stridulous and at times very labored, was quiet and natural. With the exception of a very mild and brief attack of asthma, accompanying an acute rhinitis with consequent nasal obstruction, which occurred about a month later, this patient has had no asthmatic symptoms since the operation. She has been able to take employment, goes out in all kinds of weather, takes no more than ordinary care of herself, and considers herself cured.

---

# ALTERATIVES IN NERVOUS DISEASES.

## By THE LATE WILLIAM F HUTCHINSON, M. D., PROVIDENCE, R. I.

(Reprinted from the *New England Medical Monthly*, August, 1890.)

Each year of my special practice in diseases of the nervous system, I grow more and more convinced that too much stress is placed upon the use of tonics and stimulants therein, and too little reliance upon drugs intended to change blood. There is a distinct limit to the former for they rapidly lose effect if continued any great length of time, and their number although large, is not sufficient to keep up a non-ending relay. It is curious how soon toleration of any one of this class of remedies is established up to immense doses, and how long it is before the system recovers so that small ones will have the primary effect I have a patient upon whom a less dose of compound elixir of cinchona than four ounces is useless, and who only feels that dose pleasantly. Every practitioner has had similar experiences, and has gone through the gamut of tonics only to turn in disgust from the shelf that holds them, in despair of finding something new.

It is in the hope of supplying this need that I wish to call attention to some of my own work in the line of nervous diseases, in which I am interested.

About two years ago a young lady came from central Maine to me suffering with an obscure disease of the spinal cord, which had prostrated her nervous system and made of a strong girl an apparently hopeless invalid. For months she had been unable to help herself from exhaustion, all functions were disturbed, and melancholia threatened.

After a few days' rest, I began the use of central galvanism systematically, and continued it for ten days. At the end of this time, in place of improvement, there was positive loss. She was weaker than at first, and it became evident that something else was called for.

She was then placed in an isolated, quiet room, with a trained nurse, and fed with my favorite mixture of equal parts of cream and Valentine's beef juice a teaspoonful every half hour. At the same time I commenced the administration of iodine, using by preference Gardner's syrup of Hydriodic Acid in ten drop doses hourly I find that this preparation is by far the best form of iodine for rapid dosing, as it is pleasant to taste and rarely, if ever, produces coryza.

In three days the girl showed improvement, and in three more was so much better that seclusion was abandoned, and the dietary enlarged to take in some solid food. The iodine was continued in drachm doses of the same syrup four times daily for another week, when Miss B. was on the high road to cure, and had commenced to taste metal plainly.

The iodine was then exchanged for Hypophosphites, a half ounce at bed time. Contrary to usual belief, I find this the most effective way of using this drug. There is a more rapid absorption going on during sleep than in waking hours, and the nervous system is more susceptible to influences of all kinds.

At the end of three weeks of the Hypophosphites, accompanied by a diet list of usual proportions, Miss B. was sufficiently well to be permitted to return home, and has since remained in fair health.

The preparation last used was also from the Gardner laboratory, and I am convinced that it is essential to have these compounds pure, a condition that does not exist in every formula on the market.

I have had a bottle of each of these remedies of this make on a shelf in my medicine closet for six months without undergoing any change, either in color, taste or therapeutical properties, and can recommend them as reliable.

All nervous diseases are either accompanied by or are the result of blood change, and will be most successfully treated by such means as will tend to restore the blood to a normal condition, and in my experience these have proven to be alteratives."

**Purpura, Sclerosis of Liver.**—Dr. J. K. Cantrell, Alton, Mo., March 4, 1893, writes: "I have just completed a cure of a case of purpura, a child two and one-half years old, and I must say that out of twenty years' practice, and I have treated some sixteen cases of purpura, some of the hemorrhagic form, I never treated one so successfully as this last one, and my success is due to syrup of Hydriodic Acid (Gardner's). I am also treating a case of sclerosis of the liver—patient improving fast; had hematemesis until he was almost dead; has not had a hemorrhage since he commenced the remedy."

# PYELITIS AND CYSTITIS.

### By W. B. FLETCHER, M. D., INDIANAPOLIS, IND.

(Reprinted from the *Charlotte Medical Journal*, N. C., November, 1894.

"T. A. A., a clerk in the United States Court came to me for examination four months ago. He is forty-seven years old, five feet five inches high, weight eighty-seven pounds. He came to me because of certain nervous symptoms which had alarmed him; although not in good health for ten years, and under the treatment of various physicians most of that time.

He had not been confined to his bed, but was able to "drag round" at his work. He said, "I do not expect to get well but my head is aching so constantly and I have such weakness in my legs that it frightens me." Upon inspection of the naked body, I found the skin roughened in patches, particularly over the chest, in spots from the size of a dime to that of your hand.

The roughness was like grease covered with fine bread crumbs, which could be removed by friction with a dry cloth. The abdomen was rather prominent, there was tenderness over the ascending and decending colon and some pain in pressure over the loins.

Ophthalmic examination showed extremely contracted pupil, which under atropia dilated fully, when the optic disk was found congested, the arteries varicose. Ophthalmoscopic examination particularly called my attention to the kidneys, as being the probable cause of his head and general nervous symptoms, and upon making chemical and microscopical investigation of the urine I found that it was loaded with pus, with epithelium from the pelvis of the kidneys, a few granular casts and a large quantity of bladder epithelium. I found on inquiring that he had to urinate about every three hours day and night, and that the urine had looked light and yellowish for several years, but the deposit was greater of late. I prescribed hot sponge baths followed by a cold wipe down and dry frictions every night. Washing the bladder with a saturated solution of boric acid every third morning, and Gardner's syrup of Hydriodic Acid before meals. The results were in one week again of two pounds in weight, a normal pupil, a clear skin, a gradual diminishing headache, a better feeling in loin and legs.

All these improvements continuing until at the end of three months he weighed 112 pounds and says he feels well, something never experienced since the close of the war. I regard the cure of this case due to the Hydriodic Acid, as its tonic alterative properties upon the sympathetic system have been so frequently demonstrated in my own practice, whenever the glandular organs were at fault or defective nutrition caused degeneration of the vaso-motor centers as in exophthalmic goitre, chronic tabes, mysentericus, etc., etc.

I prefer Gardner's preparations to any I have used as being less liable to produce irritation of the stomach or cause headache as a great many other preparations do."

---

"Hydriodic Acid syrup is a very pleasant and certainly an efficient way of giving iodine in chronic broncho-plumonary affections. It should not be used if discolored; one of the best preparations is that made by R. W. Gardner, of New York, of unchangeable syrup of Hydriodic Acid. It renders excellent service in asthma, chronic induration of the lungs after pneumonia, pleuritic exudations, and in some skin diseases." "*Materia Medica, Pharmacology and Therapeutics*," Shoemaker, vol. 2, page 706, (1891).

# AUTUMNAL CATARRH.

## By S. C. MARTIN, M. D..

Prof. Dermatology and Hygiene, Barnes Medical College, St. Louis, Mo.

(Reprinted from the *St. Louis Medical Era*, September, 1894.)

This disease is not, as its usual designation implies, strictly an autumnal affection. It occurs oftener in the fall of the year than at other seasons, but may be encountered in any month of the year. Nor is it produced, as formerly supposed exclusively by the pollen of certain grasses, although this is probably among the stimuli that may excite an attack where the predisposing causes are in full operation. The fact that the disease is more common in the larger cities, where the air is laden with a variety of impurities from innumerable sources, and men, who are exposed to these agencies more than women, are the most frequent victims, weakens very much the theory of pollen as a principal factor in its etiology. A neurasthenic constitution, supported by imprudent habits, often furnishes the soil for its development. It is essentially an irritation or inflammation of the mucosa of the eyes, nasal and air passages, often attended by profuse secretion from these parts, and asthmatic manifestations. It is easily distinguished from other forms of asthma by its anatomical and pathological characteristics, rarely, if ever, appearing at night, while spasmodic asthma as rarely appears in the day time. Heredity probably has its bearing on this disease, as the writer has noticed some connection of this affection with a tubercular diathesis, having discovered frequent deaths from tuberculosis in the families of those whom he has treated for hay fever. The neurotic influence seems to be an indispensable factor, otherwise the disease would not be developed on about the same day of the same month for several years successively, as often happens, and be produced by even the sight of artificial flowers, as is well authenticated by various observers. Malarial influences undoubtedly often have much to do with the development of hay fever, as in several instances it yielded in the writer's observation to large and repeated doses of quinine. This disease is marked by its sudden onset and excessive sensitiveness of the nasal passages to any unusual irritant. Unless rigid treatment is enforced or the patient transferred to other environments, the disease may continue for several weeks, and after subsiding leave him in a debilitated condition from which he may not recover for months. The same difficulty that stands in the way of a thorough understanding of the underlaying causes of hay fever also embarrasses its treatment. As a general thing a change of locality and surroundings of the patient is indicated. If he lives in the city he should go to the country, and if he lives in the country, should be sent to some place of improved sanitary environment. Any inherited or acquired infirmities should be eliminated. The nervous system is generally shattered and should be invigorated. To this end we may have recourse to strychnine, arsenic, and phosphorus, in some suitable form. Sometimes a trip, when it is possible, on the sea or lakes will be all that is required. If the secretions are very profuse, atropine will have a good effect. If the nasal passages are very irritable or sensitive, some authors advise superficial cauterization with chromic or carbolic acid. For temporary relief the writer has never found anything equal to hydrochlorate of cocaine by spray or insufflation, of the strength of three or four per cent.—the amount during twenty-four hours should not exceed one-third of a grain, and should never be entrusted to the patient's judgment, but used only under the observation of the physician. By carrying out this rule the risk of accidents and habits that might prove disastrous to the patient are avoided. For a long time iodine, in combination with the alkaline bases, has been used with more or less favorable results in all forms of asthma, especially of a reflex character. The objection to the use of the old preparations is due to their irritating effects on the alimentary canal. as well as to their acrid, disagreeable taste. In hay asthma, to be followed by satisfactory results, large doses are sometimes necessary, and it is not often they are tolerated,

The great value of iodine as an alterative and its adaptability to a wide range of diseases, has stimulated pharmaceutical talent and brought into use a preparation that possesses all the virtures of the old preparations without any of their objectionable qualities—we refer to the "syrup of Hydriodic Acid," manufactured by Mr. R. W. Gardner, of New York. The writer has been using this preparation for several years in all those pathological conditions where iodine is indicated with uniformly satisfactory results, more especially in asthma and goitre of a hypertrophic character. The result of its use in the treatment of hay asthma will appear in the following clinical cases:

CASE I. Mr. G., aged forty-five years, called at my office June 5, 1893, complaining of headache, nasal irritation, with profuse discharge from nasal and air passages, and asthmatic accompaniments. Had suffered from same trouble about same time of the year for several years. Had never obtained relief before the advent of heavy frosts. We sprayed nasal passages with cocaine hydrochlorate and prescribed two teaspoonfuls of "syrup of Hydriodic Acid." (Gardner) three times a day before each meal. Improvement immediately followed, and in two weeks patient was entirely cured. Advised the use of Hydriodic Acid two weeks preceding attack. The patient has up to this time, which is more than a year, had no return of the disease.

CASE 2. Mr. M., presented himself at office August 2, 1893, with a clearly established case of hay fever; had suffered for years during summer months, always at the same season of the year; had never received more than temporary relief from treatment. We prescribed cocaine insufflations and a dessertspoonful of syrup of Hydriodic Acid three times a day, before meals. Improvement promptly resulted, as in first case, and in ten days was entirely free from trouble. Advised use of same remedy two weeks preceeding next looked-for attack. The patient has been under our observation for over a year, with no reappearance of the disease.

CASE 3. Mrs. S. presented herself August 15, 1893, with marked symptoms of hay fever. Having discovered malarial features, we prescribed quinine, which relieved her very much, but did not entirely end the trouble. We ordered cocaine. It has promptly yielded under the sprays and the syrup of Hydriodic Acid in teaspoonful doses three times a day. In seven days patient was restored to her usual health, and up to this time, which is over a year, has had no return of the disease. In this case we advised resumption of treatment before expected reappearance of disease, as in former cases. In all the use we have made of this preparation we have never noticed iodism or any other unpleasant effects. While its pleasant taste, with most patients, is an important advantage it possesses over all other preparations of similar therapeutic value.

---

# SEVEN CASES OF FIBROID TUMOR, SUCCESSFULLY TREATED BY SYRUP OF HYDRIODIC ACID.

By JAMES J. TERHUNE, M. D., BROOKLYN, N. Y.

(Reprinted from the *New England Medical Monthly*, December, 1894.)

Mrs. V. B. had been complaining for a long time, a year or more, with pelvic pain, backache, but persistently refused examination and treatment. At last was taken down with severe pains and fever to such an extent as to necessitate medical attention. The first examination was made by myself and E. S. Bunker, M. D., late Professor of Obstetrics, Long Island College Hospital, in consultation; diagnosis was plain, subserous fibroid tumor, (multiple.)

In speaking of the treatment, the thought occurred to me that Hydriodic Acid would be serviceable. We therefore prescribed Gardner's syrup of Hydriodic Acid, a teaspoonful three times a day, and were very much gratified with the results, which were far beyond our expectations. The patient has fully recovered her usual health and strength, and has had no recurrence of the pains or other bad symptoms which she formerly had, and has remained so for a period of fully five years.

The result of treatment is not expected to remove the tumors, but to shrink them up and thus render them inert.

Case No. Two. Mrs. F., over forty years of age, had been troubled with extreme flowing, which greatly emaciated her. At last was taken to her bed with severe pains, and quite severe floodings. An examination was made, which revealed multiple sub-serous fibroid tumors, two of which were as large as an orange. Tamponed her, relieved the pain by opiates, and put her on syrup of Hydriodic Acid. The result of treatment was fully as beneficial as in case No. one.

Case No. Three. Mrs. T., aged about forty-two years. The condition of this case was similar to No. two. There were three or four tumors in this case, two of them anteriorly, which were large, pressed forcibly upon the bladder, produced pain in the bladder and some cystitis.

This patient was also examined by Dr. Bunker in consultation with me, and the results in cases Nos. one and three, were also verified by him. Under the treatment of syrup of Hydriodic Acid, the woman has been brought to a perfectly comfortable condition. She had but one relapse, about two years after the first treatment, due to extra work and fatigue consequent upon removing into a newly purchased house.

Previous to treatment she was unable to go out or exercise at all for a year or more, and after three weeks' treatment was able to go about as she pleased.

Case No. Four. Mrs. Y. came to my office, very anæmic, had been under the care of physicians about two years; more than half of the time she had been flooding more or less. At last an operation was advised and time fixed for it. Her mother requested her to call and see me for my opinion before having it done. I advised her to wait and see the result of treatment before submitting to the operation.

Examination revealed the uterus firmly fixed by sub-serous fibroid multiple tumors; also, protruding from the os, was a sub-mucous fibroid with quite large base; painted the same with tincture iodine compound, and placed her upon syrup of Hydriodic Acid, with opiates to relieve pain. When she next called, in about two weeks' time, she stated that she had ceased flooding and felt better than she had for two years. Her next two monthly periods were five weeks apart, with but three days' flowing, as she used to be before she was troubled with the tumors. She is still under treatment and tumors diminishing in size, with the sub-mucous one becoming more protruding and pedunculated.

I had three other cases which were progressing finely, but being office patients, and non-residents of the city, they have passed from under my notice. I could not, therefore, give as good and as satisfactory a statement of the results, as in the preceding four, who are members of my regular families.

---

# KIDNEY PAIN.

By WM. C. WILE, A. M., M. D., LL. D., DANBURY, CONN.

(Reprinted from *New England Medical Monthly*, July, 1894.)

In the treatment of every case of pyelitis and renal colic, the practitioner has a great deal of difficulty in controlling the pain in the kidneys. The editor of the *Monthly* has been a sufferer for years from a gouty condition, which manifested itself about four times a year in acute attacks of renal colic. In the intervals between these attacks the pain in the kidney was not so severe as during an acute paroxysm of the disease. Still it was constant, aggravating, and often sleep-destroying, especially following a day of hard work.  My attention was called to the use of syrup of  Hydriodic Acid in kidney pains by Dr. F. King, of New York city, who had been a sufferer from the same trouble.  We did not try it, however, until it was ordered by Dr. L. Bolton Bangs, the eminent authority on Genito-Urinary Diseases, of New York city, under whose skillful care the writer was for over a year.  The effect of this remedy was astounding.  Only two day's administration of teaspoonful doses (which were subsequently increased to two teaspoonfuls) relieved the pain almost entirely, and it would return only on occasions of broken rest and great fatigue from brain wear and tear.  It is a splendid antiseptic to the genito-urinary tract, and we are confident that as a kidney pain reliever it is simply head and shoulders over anything else that we  know of. This result has been confirmed a great many times in different people and by different practitioners.  The preparation that we always use is that of R. W.  Gardner, of 158 William street, New York city—one of the best chemists in the United States.

---

# ŒDEMA OF GLOTTIS—CHRONIC INTERSTITIAL NEPHRITIS—TERTIARY SYPHILIS.

### By L. A. TURNBULL, M. D., Visiting Physician.

#### (Clinical Report from St. Louis Female Hospital.)

H. E., female; aged 55; widow; admitted June 22, 1894.
June 23.  Family history cannot be ascertained.
Previous history:  Has had several diseases peculiar to infancy and childhood. General health good.  Twenty-nine years ago had a hard chancre on right labia majora —about three months later the secondary eruption appeared; a year after primary lesion had iritis; a year later necrosis of nasal eminence and spine of frontal bone, followed by necrosis of nasal bone and palate process of superior maxillary bone.
Habits:  Excessively alcoholic, after infection for three or four years.
Hygienic surroundings, poor.
Present trouble began about seven years ago; an occasional attack of asthma, which became more frequent; had œdema of lower extremities; about this time secured medical treatment and managed to do her work until seven weeks ago, when her trouble became greatly aggravated; continued mapiratory dyspnœa; was unable to assume the recumbent position at night; pain in cardiac region; headache; loss of appetite; weak and exhausted.
Present condition:  Patient is poorly nourished (anæmic); the skin is cool and dry; tongue is very pale, moist and clean; no appetite; bowels generally constipated; pulse is rapid (110 per minute); poor volume and tension; temperature normal;  respiration rapid (30 per minute), short and incomplete.
Physical examination:  Face has a worn and anxious expression; is wrinkled and pinched; eyes protrude and stare; skin is dirty-looking, tawny, dry, and has no luster. The hair is thin; the epidermis exfoliates excessively; patient is despondent, nervous and fretful.  The general condition indicates depression of vital forces; lower extremities are œdematous—pit on pressure and exhibit marks of former ulcerative lesions; small depression over the sight of former necrosis of frontal bone, also on right side of the nose; almost all of the hard palate has ulcerated away; also part of the soft palate (with uvula).
Inspirations are harsh, loud and short over the larger bronchias; otherwise lungs are normal; area of heart dullness increased—visible impulse increased—downward and slightly outward; patient experiences pain when this region is percussed.  The sounds are very clear and sharp; the first sound is prolonged; a clink is very pronounced just to the right of the apex beat.  Liver dullness increased; spleen enlarged.

Urinalysis: Specific gravity 1030; acid reaction; reddish-yellow color; 1 per cent. albumen; no sugar; quantity greatly decreased.
Diagnosis. Glottic œdema; chronic interstitial nephritis; tertiary syphilis.
Treatment. Nitro-glycerine 3 times a day; magnesia sulph. (as required) once a day; syrup Hydriodic Acid (Gardner's) teaspoonful 4 times daily. Patient is improving.

## IODINE INTERNALLY AS AN ALTERATIVE.

### By I. N. LOVE, M. D.

Vice-President American Medical Association.

(Reprinted from the *Medical Mirror*, St. Louis, June, 1894.)

Since the days of Coindet, Brera, Lugol, and Manson, the medical profession has been fully impressed with the value of the internal administration of iodine for its alterative effects. Every practitioner of any experience has seen numerous cases where various tumefactions, glandular enlargements, and even what seemed to be tubercular and carcinomatous conditions, were greatly improved and seemingly cured by this remedy.

Iodine is supposed, like chloride of sodium, to be one of the natural constituents of the human body. Given in medicinal doses it is of great value. From clinical observation extending over a long period of years, I am convinced that it acts beneficially chiefly in that it is a special stimulant to that function of the body by which all of its parts are undergoing continuous disintegration and renewal. It stimulates and assists in the exchange of products, aiding assimilation, its elimination, and the metabolism of tissues; in other words, under administration there is a stimulation of the activities of the secretory system of the glands. Digestion is thus improved and nutrition is encouraged; waste products are more rapidly carried away, and tone and vigor result.

Knowing the sluggish state of the system in the so-called scrofulous condition (that indefinite expression covering a multitude of sins as it does; sins that may be of remote ancestry); and in those conditions dependent upon later individual sins upon the part of the victim, coming under the head of specific diseases, where an even greater stasis upon the part of the secretory organs is present; and in that indefinite state known as the rheumatic, which is after all better expressed by the term lymphostasis, or a stasis or the lymph vessels,—iodine is the ideal remedy.

For long the problem has been how best to give this remedy. Given direct in the form of tincture largely diluted, it soon becomes an irritant to the stomach. It is often given in combination with mercury and potassium, the iodide of potassium being the favorite form. But how often do we find the stomach rebels against it; how often do all of the mucous membranes of the body become riotous and resent the intrusion of the remedy.

For years, with children particularly, in whom digestion is easily impaired, where agreeableness and pleasantness cut so large a figure in medicine, and even with adults I have found no form of administering iodine so satisfactory as the syrup of Hydriodic Acid. To R. W. Gardner, of New York, is the profession indebted for the perfection of this form for administration.

The iodide of hydrogen (Hydriodic Acid) causes no irritation because it is an acid solution which does not interfere with digestion. It is as agreeable to the taste as lemon syrup, and will invariably be accepted freely by the most delicate female and young children; and by the way, the average man has just as much regard for his palate as those of the supposed weaker side of the world; so we do not go far wrong if

76

we give them their iodine in an agreeable, acceptable form. It may be used without intermission. It produces no depression, no indigestion, no irritation; and invariably where I have found idiosyncrasies against the use of iodide of potassium, where catarrhal and other disagreeable disturbances of the mucous membrane were aroused, the Gardner syrup of Hydriodic Acid has uniformly been well tolerated.

Since the introduction to the medical profession of the syrup of Hydriodic Acid by Mr. Gardner, fifteen years ago, I have constantly used the remedy, and have never had occasion to regret it. I should as soon think of permitting a druggist to substitute tincture of marigold for the green tincture of digitalis, when I desire to reduce the rapidity of the heart's action, with the question of life and death involved, as to allow any druggist to substitute any other syrup of Hydriodic Acid in place of that of R. W. Gardner. The medical profession is under special obligations to Mr. Gardner for his careful, skillful, scientific work as a chemist in this direction, and it should endorse him by its support, knowing that good results can be expected to follow the use of his preparation.